THE FOREST REMINDS US WHO WE ARE

THE FOREST REMINDS US WHO WE ARE

*Connecting to the
Living Medicine
of Wild Plants*

Seán Pádraig O'Donoghue

North Atlantic Books
Berkeley, California

Published by
North Atlantic Books
Berkeley, California

Cover photo © gettyimages.com/Rán An/EyeEm
Cover design by John Yates
Book design by Happenstance Type-O-Rama

Printed in the United States of America

The Forest Reminds Us Who We Are: Connecting to the Living Medicine of Wild Plants is sponsored and published by North Atlantic Books, an educational nonprofit based in Berkeley, California, that collaborates with partners to develop cross-cultural perspectives, nurture holistic views of art, science, the humanities, and healing, and seed personal and global transformation by publishing work on the relationship of body, spirit, and nature.

North Atlantic Books' publications are available through most bookstores. For further information, visit our website at www.northatlanticbooks.com or call 800-733-3000.

Library of Congress Cataloging-in-Publication Data

Names: O'Donoghue, Seán Pádraig, 1974– author.
Title: The forest reminds us who we are : connecting to the living medicine
   of wild plants / Seán Pádraig O'Donoghue.
Description: Berkeley, California : North Atlantic Books, [2021] | Includes
   bibliographical references and index. | Summary: "A guide book for
   tapping into the medicinal power of wild plants for recovering and
   maintaining spiritual, emotional, and mental wellbeing"— Provided by
   publisher.
Identifiers: LCCN 2020056415 (print) | LCCN 2020056416 (ebook) | ISBN
   9781623175702 (paperback) | ISBN 9781623175719 (epub)
Subjects: LCSH: Medicinal plants. | Medicinal plants—Identification. |
   Wild plants, Edible—Therapeutic use.
Classification: LCC QK99.A1 O325 2021 (print) | LCC QK99.A1 (ebook) | DDC
   581.6/34—dc23
LC record available at https://lccn.loc.gov/2020056415
LC ebook record available at https://lccn.loc.gov/2020056416

1 2 3 4 5 6 7 8 9 KPC 26 25 24 23 22 21

for

Mo Bhanríon Fiáin

with deep gratitude for the braiding
of the wild roads we walk

ACKNOWLEDGMENTS

I give thanks first of all to the plants, the land, the water, and my ancestors, human and wild, and then to my Beloved, to whom this book is dedicated and who encouraged and inspired me throughout its writing, even through the long Maine winter in the midst of a pandemic.

This book would not exist without the encouragement of Tim McKee and the support and assistance of Gillian Hamel, the editors I have been working with at North Atlantic Books. Thank you for believing in this project. Thank you also to Jennifer Eastman at North Atlantic for smoothing the rough edges of this book, helping the ideas woven through it to find their best expression.

My dear friend and teacher Cornelia Benavidez pored over many drafts of this manuscript, offering a keen eye and wonderful suggestions and insights. She is also a deep well of wisdom and inspiration and my living connection to her teachers, Victor and Cora Anderson, whose work and teachings, along with Cornelia's own, have transformed my life in such beautiful and profound ways, though I never met Victor and Cora while they were alive.

My mother, Sandy Donahue, helped to edit some of the early drafts of some of the material in this book. She also introduced me to poetry, myth, and folklore and fed me my first wild foods. My father, Brian Donahue, taught me who the O'Donoghues were and are, and taught me to be proud of my Irish ancestry. He and my brother, Ryan, and my sister, Shannon, have been wonderfully encouraging throughout this process.

Crystal Murphy helped edit some early drafts of a few of these chapters as well.

Alicia Crockett believed in this book and in me even when I didn't. Thank you.

Many of the ideas that gave rise to this book found their earliest expression in articles I wrote for *Plant Healer* magazine and at the conferences organized by its editors, Kiva Rose Hardin and Jesse Wolf Hardin. I am deeply grateful for the kindness, inspiration, and insight they have both provided over the years, and for their deep commitment to the healing and re-enchantment of the world.

Dr. Mitch Bebel Stargrove and Dr. Lori Stargrove shared many nights of conversation with me around their kitchen table, with other eclectic thinkers sometimes joining us. These conversations echo through parts of this book.

Sage Maurer helped me find my way to Ireland and introduced me to its sacred wells, and Alan Cooke helped me connect more deeply with the spirit of the land—and introduced me to the work of John Moriarty.

Dr. Kenneth Proefrock's lectures helped me rediscover my childhood love of science and understand neurochemistry, phytochemistry, and their implications for consciousness.

Nick Walker's writing about neurodiversity, neurodivergence, and the Autistic mind and experience helped me understand my own neurobiology.

Mischa Schuler introduced me to herbalism.

I have learned so much about the lives and medicine of wild plants from so many herbalists over the years. I am grateful to everyone who has ever sat with me and spoke about plants. There are three herbalists whose guidance I especially want to give thanks for:

Margi Flint taught me how to read the body and how to meet people where they are and walk with them on their healing journeys.

Matthew Wood taught me how to read energetic patterns and how to understand the unique medicine and personality of each plant.

Stephen Harrod Buhner taught me how to listen directly to the voices of the plants and how to live, speak, and write from my heart.

All three of them have shown tremendous kindness and generosity in good times and hard times and have my endless gratitude.

Go raibh míle maith agat.

CONTENTS

FOREWORD

Entering a book, an unimagined yet somehow clear perception opens, and a sense of familiar experience arises. The objective and subjective flow back and forth into each other as past memory, immediate sensation, and future visions reveal patterns of emergence grounded in knowing within relationship.

After many years of observing Seán in his glories and travails, I see here a story of a storyteller being told. He shares synchronicities and revelations while weaving history, poetry, plants, and life sciences throughout the events and relationships of his experience. As Seán has matured in his storytelling, he has achieved a dynamic equilibrium between oral tradition and written presentation. The expanded openness that Seán generates when speaking is accessed and induced by these words of magick.

Having knowing Seán for many years, I've often felt a shared comfort and discomfort with Seán, a vague sense of familiarity, of us being revolutionaries together or, more poignantly, being two heretical Catholic priests of long ago, an Irishman and a Pole, pondering more ancient memories in involuntary seclusion. We found ourselves natural allies engaged in social medicine and applied natural therapies toward creating regenerative cultures and birthing a Nu Aeon every day. Loving the ancient past, especially before Empire, Seán reveals visions and shares deeply felt experiences that are the daily reality of our process of co-creating healthy futures in alignment with Gaia. Rooted in our ancestors, honoring the lands in which we live, and manifesting the Art of Living, together—this is *the* Work of these times.

The presence, tone, and voice of this book are vividly Seán's, as reflected in his approach and improvisation, and this extends the content itself. The working vision framing this book is rooted in an ancient three-worlds model and expands into ecology, complexity theory, bioregional reintegration, and postbinary culture. Seán thrives on igniting enthusiasm in each of us as he demonstrates that science can be mythic and that the mythic is immediate and omnipresent. This is more than an "herb book," because in it we experience plant medicine through relationships and observations of living networks. While proudly identifying as neurodivergent, Seán makes no claim to exclusive access to hidden secrets. He serves as a poet, storyteller, and guide, as well as a Gaian herbalist modeling mythically informed embodied awareness as a postbinary visionary activist.

Seán is an exemplar of a modern successor to the *Draoi* of pre-Christian Ireland, weaving magick and science, poetry and physiology with plants and charms, thus creating radical possibilities. As Carl Jung exhorts, learning the traditions of other cultures can enrich us, but we gain power and insight from aligning with the deep roots of our own heritages, particularly, in this case, the folk traditions of Europe. Known by specific indigenous names in each culture, they are distinguished by initiated lineages, offer a panoply of medicine and magick, and are the ones who provided medical care for most folks throughout history. Looking back, it becomes all too evident that there is a big hole in our medical history. If classical physicians of the past were treating only the elites, who was providing medical care for most of the population, especially in the rural areas, hamlets, and small towns where most people lived? Hidden between the "educated" physicians and the unnamed of family self-care, they would gather and prescribe herbs, use enchanted psalms, counsel with astrology and divination, clear curses, invoke mates, and help with a variety of problems of family, home, and farm.

I smile when I see the excitement of discovery in the eyes of students and practitioners of natural medicine about the non-physician lineages of medical practice in premodern Europe. They often say that they feel reconnected to a deep part of their own history and to medicine's possibilities, which embody long-lost "relatives of blood and bone, of vision and service." I see many who aspire to a professional drawing from both the classical physician and the mythic witch/shaman, as well as from the old wives and medicine people. They do so in order to express an authentic contemporary synthesis realized in moments of synchronistic certainty but, as yet, not fully imagined. In this work, Seán demonstrates that this can be done, playing upon the emerging edge where the outer intervention of medicine dances with the inner art of self-healing.

Seán goes deep. Seán soars.
Seán suffers. Seán celebrates.
Seán smiles silently in bliss.
Seán is a Heathen,
Fear Feasa,
Witch,
WortCharmer,
Cunning Man,
Bard and—
rEvolutionary.

If you seek a natural-therapies recipe book to see what you might take for your headache, gut pain, or insomnia, in this book you may find exactly what you need, yet maybe not in the way you expected. However, once you have shared some spacetime with Seán and his words, you may never feel the same way as you walk through the forest and fields. Many books offer knowledge in what medicine *does,* but only a few show us the *how* of catalyzing healing, transformation born of experience, and deep relationship.

Whether inviting Devil's Club or Damiana, mycelial interplay or bear magick—or offering a juicy poem or gem of physiology—Seán moves the dance into unexplored perceptual territory embodying Mysteries. Yet the wisdom shared here is of a journey taken together, even if we each experience completely different plants, places, or events as we read. Seán activates the reader as if through gnostic *shaktipat*, spreading seeds of spontaneous recognition and offering medicine for each and all. Revealing his deepest aspirations for and dedication to Healing, Justice, and Peace, Seán challenges himself and the reader to fully engage in the experiment of socially conscious compassionate engagement. This experiment embodies manifesting Gandhian self-reliance, mutual aid ethics, and Heathen embodiments on the edge of civilization.

Seán is a *permissionary,* reminding us that we always have permission to be true to our self-knowing and self-creating. He invites us into experiential gnostic learning by telling us to just take a few drops daily, and see, feel, and heal. As befits a skillful Satyagraha TruthForce Warrior, Seán enters our world by invitation, catalyzes a latent potency toward self-healing and reorganization, and, smiling, silently steps aside as the emergent process unfolds. The method and content of his transmissions remind us to stay attuned to the mythopoetic wellspring of our deep being. This is the source of healing, connection, and renewal. Healing is not primarily about medicine or herbs or even about symptoms improving—rather, healing comes as we deepen our perception, transform our experience, and come to peace with life as it is.

All medicine ultimately relies on self-healing, and in these times, we are healing within ourselves and in our relationships and behaviors as we align with Gaia, of which we are all part. The coherent life flow moving through this planet as a dynamic living system is the same as the vitality and self-organizing processes within our bodies. The metaphor and the biology overlap and enrich each other. This is the rich forest into which we venture with Seán, through many eras and at many scales of becoming.

To quote Seán, "deepening of awareness is a fundamental part of the healing process."

Healing ripples long after medicine treats. This book teaches and activates the reader on all levels, nourishing the Root, connecting information through relationships and patterns, and inspiring the HeartMind. As with any journey, the experiences along the way enrich life afterward.

Enjoy, and

.be well,

Dr. Mitch Stargrove

Mitchell Bebel Stargrove, ND, LAc earned his BA in history and government from Oberlin College in 1979, his acupuncture diploma from Oregon College of Oriental Medicine (OCOM) in 1987, and his naturopathic degree from National College of Naturopathic Medicine (NCNM) in 1988. He is licensed as an acupuncturist and naturopathic physician in Oregon and practices with Dr. Lori Beth Stargrove at A WellSpring of Natural Health, Inc., in Beaverton. Since 1990 he has taught the history of medicine at OCOM (to present) and NCNM (1990–1993). Dr. Stargrove is the editor and coauthor of *Herb, Nutrient, and Drug Interactions: Clinical Implications and Therapeutic Strategies* (MosbyElsevier, 2008). He coordinated the development of and compiled the acupuncture section for the *Integrative BodyMind Information System* (IBIS), the pioneering multidisciplinary electronic encyclopedia for practitioners of integrative medicine and natural therapeutics (published in 1993), and is editor-in-chief of *InteractionsGuide* and *ChoicesForHealth: IBIS*. In addition, he is chief medical officer of MedicineWorks (https://medicineworks.com), a division of Health Resources Unlimited, Inc., as well as a founder and board member of the Alchemical Medicine Research and Teaching Association (AMRTA). Dr. Stargrove is lead history editor of and a contributing author to the text *Foundations of Naturopathic Medicine* (in press) and lead author and co-editor of *Naturopathic Medicine History and Professional Formation Timeline* (in press). In August 2012, the American Association of Naturopathic Physicians presented him with the *Vis Medicatrix Naturae* award in recognition of his activities as a "naturopathic physician who represents the healing power of nature as demonstrated through work, life and community service." In 2015, Dr. Stargrove was invited to be a founding member of the Naturopathic Council of Elders. During 2015, he and a team of community members founded CascadiaFire, a bioregional service organization that celebrates sacred fire circle gatherings. Drs. Mitch and Lori teach therapeutic strategies in person-centered collaborative care, host the GaiaStar Temple, and coordinate the Blue Lotus Mystery School as they explore embodied methods of self-healing, cocreativity, and respectful living. The Oregon Association of Naturopathic Physicians and National University of Natural Medicine honored Dr. Stargrove with the Living Legend Award in December 2017.

And see ye not that bonny road

That winds about the fernie brae?

That is the road to fair Elfland

Where thou and I this night maun gae

—CHILD BALLAD 37, "THOMAS RHYMER"

INTRODUCTION

The Wound Is Where the Healing Comes

L ike many children, I grew up knowing viscerally that the world was
alive.

Being Autistic, I held onto that knowledge longer than most people do in
this culture.

Autistic brains create more synapses than other brains, and those synapses proliferate in nonlinear ways. Hence, our brains are likely to observe
patterns and connections that others miss—and rebel against accepting
structures that do not conform to our experience of reality. We also take in
more sensory information than most people, which can be sublime or excru-
ciating, or both, depending on our environment.

Our difficulty accepting hierarchies of being that do not follow logic and
our tendency to pick up on the emotions and sensations of other beings in
our environment imbues Autistic people with a certain innate and intuitive
animism. We empathize with beings whom our culture does not recognize
as people—Whales, Cedars, Stars, Stones, Sentient Machines.

This perception puts us further out of step with a culture that is already
uncomfortable with the differences in the ways we move, think, and speak (or,

in some cases, don't speak). Childhood tends to be a lonely time for a lot of Autistic people, and it was for me. I found my solace in folklore and fantasy novels that spoke of other worlds that seemed hauntingly familiar—and in the woods.

There was a trail behind our house, through a swampy forest filled with Skunk Cabbage that led to a field of tall grass, Crab Apple, and Sumac that I called the Secret Hideout. Everything there had a strange luminosity that reminded me of the once and future worlds that called to me from behind the impenetrable veil of history.

I also knew that this world was in danger from people who did not understand that it was alive and who were willing to destroy it to get what they wanted. At nine, I could explain the dangers of nuclear winter and acid rain and was writing poetry about endangered species. At ten, I took a break from walking around the playground writing stories in my head to stand by the fence holding up homemade poster-board signs about Reagan's nuclear arms buildup for the passing cars to see.

Asthma, a lack of coordination, and trouble navigating social situations made sports and gym class a nightmare for me, and I developed the sense that my body was broken and that sensation and emotion were enemies. Sugar and starches became effective tools for shutting down perception.

As I grew older, the fear remained and grew into outrage, but my sense of connection to the living world I wanted to save was fading into a mere abstraction. I spent my twenties and early thirties blockading weapons plants, documenting human rights atrocities, and reading, writing, and scheming about revolution. But no matter what I did, it never seemed commensurate with the level of suffering and destruction I was witnessing in the world, so I felt inadequate and kept trying to push myself further.

I was living a life in which I was deeply disconnected from my body—a lifetime of body shame overlapping with the remnants of a theology of martyrdom. I was struggling with asthma, depression, and insulin resistance that had me on the verge of diabetes. I was working more than full time as a human rights activist for a small organization in Bangor, Maine, and viewed my body as a broken thing that mattered only as a vehicle for resisting the status quo, which seemed like the empire of modern myth. After a decade and a half of activism, I was feeling the futility of it all. So I threw myself into a war zone.

I went to Oaxaca, in southern Mexico, at a time when the city was occupied by military police who had come to crush an uprising. My heart was broken open by the strength of the people I met hiding in church basements, who had lived through horrors, and by the people I met in the mountains, who spoke of the land and the Corn as shaping their sense of who they were, which revealed exactly the empty place inside me from which the hunger for meaning arose.

The night that I came back, for some reason I thought it was a good idea to go to a dinner party in Boston, something I would tend to view as nightmarish on the best of days, let alone when blown wide open. There was one person there whose presence felt different than anyone else's. When we finally spoke, she told me that she was an herbalist and began to speak of listening to the plants and of helping people regain connection with their own bodies. I was intrigued.

She called me a few weeks later, on New Year's Day, when I was sick with bronchitis. After we hung up, she called me back and said she had been listening to my breathing and knew the plant who could help me—"She has a bright yellow flower and a deep, resinous root and moves what we hold on to in our lungs. Her name is Elecampane."

When I took my first drops of Elecampane tincture that afternoon, I felt breath enter me deeply and experienced the unraveling of the story that my body was broken and could not be healed. I went walking in the snowy woods with my dog, breathing in the scent of Fir and Spruce and Pine, feeling my chest open wider and new life stir within me.

In the coming weeks, breath brought me more into my body, and I discovered how much I loved lifting heavy things. As weightlifting came into my life, my body started craving deeper nourishment, and following my intuition, I started shifting how I ate, how I moved, and how I breathed.

Then, everything collapsed—an on-again, off-again romance that had broken open my heart finally came to an end at the same time that the funding ran out for my job. Believing that any path was better than the one I was on, I went walking in the Bangor City Forest and prayed to get lost.

My eyes were drawn to the *Usnea* lichen that had fallen to the ground in the last rainstorm, its threads like the hair and beard of the wild Green Man of the forest. I followed the fallen *Usnea* until I found myself standing in a ring of Spruces I have never seen before. I closed my eyes and saw *Usnea*'s tendrils reaching into the cracked places in my heart.

I spent most of the following summer wandering through forest and field, listening deeply to the plants, and reading herb books at night.

When autumn came, I returned to the city, taking a job helping military families tell the stories of how the war in Iraq had devastated their lives. The wells of grief at the center of their hearts and mine seemed bottomless. I began to feel overwhelm and despair again. So in the spring I went to the White Mountains of New Hampshire to listen to the forest.

By the third day of my vision quest, fasting alone in the forest, just above a stream flowing into the Pemigewasset River, it was all I could do to stumble to the edge of the ten-foot stone circle that marked the boundary of my world.

Just beyond that border, I saw a fallen hemlock branch covered in lichen—and among the lichens, a patch of *Usnea* that seemed to glow with a pale light. To protect the trees that it grows on from infection, *Usnea* produces antibacterial and antifungal compounds that also serve as powerful medicine for humans and other animals.

From somewhere inside my chest, I heard the voice of the lichen speaking, telling me that the lichen would often grow in the places where the tree was wounded, that the wounds themselves called forth the medicine. A song began to rise inside me:

The wound is where the healing comes,
The wound is where the change begins!
Break on open and feel again,
Break on open and dream again,
Break on open and grow again,
Break on open and live again!

As I sang out loud, cycling through the chant again and again, questions and contradictions I had been struggling with began to resolve themselves.

Central was the conflict I felt between the political work I had dedicated my adult life to up to then and the healing work that I had been powerfully drawn to in recent years. More and more, it had been working to bring people together with plants that could support the healing of their bodies, minds, and spirits that had made me feel most alive. But strong voices inside me had been insisting that I had a responsibility to be part of political and cultural transformation.

That dichotomy fell away. I thought of the people who had come into my life and the pain they were living with—veterans, torture survivors, military families, refugees. And if—as *Usnea* was telling me—"the wound is where the change begins," then by coming to know the nature of those wounds, I would also come to know the wild, living medicines that could transform the culture that wounded them, healing hearts and healing worlds.

This book is my best attempt to translate and share what I have learned from people and plants and Gods and ancestors in the decade since. May it open the way for more people to allow the forest to remind them who they are.

HEALING IN
OUR LIVING WORLD

Healing is the process of life moving through us come into its fullest and most authentic expression. My Irish ancestors spoke of health as a Salmon swimming through the oceans of the Great World that contains all worlds and then into the rivers and streams of our own lives.

Treatment (the amelioration of symptoms) and cure (the elimination of symptoms) are significantly different goals and outcomes than healing. Herbalist Peter Conway says that the difference between being cured and being healed is that you can die healed, an insight he attributes to the late homeopath Dr. Edward Bach, creator of the Bach Flower Essences. To die healed is to die while being in right relation with all things in your inner world and your outer worlds. That can happen only in a context where we recognize and experience the rest of the world as alive.

We cannot come into this full expression of who we are without allowing our consciousness to fully enter and fill our bodies. Once we are fully embodied, we experience ourselves as the animals we are—animals whose senses are attuned to the pheromones of other creatures, the scent of rain on soil, roads of inspiration on the Milky Way, and the electrical charge and buzz of the aurora borealis. We recognize them as signs of that our kin are near.

Contemporary neurobiology tells us that, as humans, we need to feel kinship with other humans for our bodies to operate in a coherent way. Less discussed is our need for other-than-human kinship. Few even make the connection that the one therapy that seems nearly universally helpful and relevant in improving the health of people suffering from the "diseases of civilization"—such as trauma, anxiety, depression, alienation, addiction, inflammation, immune dysfunction, hormonal dysregulation, and cancer—is simply walking in a forest.

Herbalists are in a unique position to facilitate healing. By guiding people in practices that connect them with plants and fungi (and with their own bodies), we can shift their relationships with themselves, their human and other-than-human relations, and the living world itself. We can do this in ways that change what it means for them to be a human embodied in this time and place, which, in turn, will change the ways their nervous and endocrine and immune systems process and respond to the world, changing everything else in their bodies in turn. But too often we fall into the trap of simply treating plants and fungi as remedies for specific ailments, echoing mainstream medicine's incomplete understanding of the nature of health and healing. My practice is rooted in seven principles:

1. Our bodies are dynamic, complex living systems, and so is the body of our world.

2. Individual, community, cultural, and ecological health are inseparable.

3. There is an intelligence inherent in these interrelated complex living systems that will tend to maintain and, when necessary, protect and restore the integrity of the system.

4. Humans need connection with other humans and with other-than-human beings to maintain optimal health.

5. Plants and fungi are not inert materials for the production of medicine, they are living beings with their own intelligences, so I seek to be in reciprocal relationship with the plants and fungi whose help I engage in healing.

6. Plants and fungi belong to themselves.

7. Beauty and wonder are ways we recognize the healthy flow of life.

1. Our bodies are dynamic, complex living systems, and so is the body of our world.

Separating mind from body and body from land, our culture has defined the land and waters as reservoirs of inert material and bodies as machines for transforming that material into wealth. Historian Silvia Federici writes (2016):

> *Capitalism was born from the separation of people from the land and its first task was to make work independent of the seasons and to lengthen the workday beyond the limits of our endurance. Generally, we stress the economic aspect of this process, the economic dependence capitalism has created on monetary relations, and its role in the formation of a wage proletariat. What we have not always seen is what the separation from the land and nature has meant for our body, which has been pauperized and stripped of the powers that pre-capitalist populations attributed to it.*

Outside the disciplines of mechanization visited on them, our bodies are capable of sensing subtle shifts in their experience of their internal ecologies—the intuitive dimensions of the pulse diagnosis come to mind—and in the world around us. Federici writes, "We know now, for instance, that the Polynesian populations used to travel the high seas at night with only their body as their compass, as they could tell from the vibrations of the waves the

9

different ways to direct their boats to the shore"—which we can gloss as "reading the pulse of the ocean," just as an herbalist or acupuncturist can map the internal terrain of the body by feeling the way blood flows past particular points on the wrist.

Bodies are constantly attuning to subtle flows within complex systems and to the ways in which everything shifts within and around them. Changes in complex systems can ultimately only be understood in terms of mapping the nature of such flows—whether through our senses, using our awareness of our own experience of embodiment as a technology of perception and investigation, or through the elaborate equations and algorithms of chaos mathematics and systems theory.

2. Individual, community, cultural, and ecological health are inseparable.

What is this thing I call a *body*, this community of cells and tissues and organs? It contains at least as many cells that we would call *viral* or *bacterial* or *fungal* as the cells we would call *Homo sapiens*. The elements that make it up are ancient—the hydrogen that combined with oxygen to form the water molecules that make up most of my body is older than the oldest stars. Yet the molecules and atoms contained in it have not been contained in it that long comparatively—in fact, the mercury and dioxin stored in my superficial fascia when my body breathed them in and couldn't figure out how to neutralize or remove them in my childhood have been part of my body far longer than any of the molecules I can identify as part of my biochemistry. If anything, this body is another habitual way matter and energy have of arranging themselves. The water that flows through my body has flowed through other human and animal bodies, as well as through soil and roots and mycelia—and my health depends on the health of everything that water flows through. The soil is the fascia of the earth and what is contained within it will be held in my fascia as well. We are the earth's rain and oceans, its fire and lightning, its minerals make up our bones. The space between our cells is like the space between stars, which is like the space between the electrons of an atom.

This is not just poetic musing. It is—as Victor Anderson, the sage and Grand Master of the Feri tradition, would say—"the way things really are."

So, who is this persona who claims to be "me"? He is a product of the interaction of the consciousness that arises within my body with the actions and expressions of the other consciousnesses around me. If I spend most of my time in the forest, my persona will take on the characteristics of a forest. If I spend most of my time among other humans, my persona will take on characteristics of the community I participate in. The health of that persona, that psyche, is dependent on the health of the community that shapes it.

3. There is an intelligence inherent in these interrelated complex living systems that will tend to maintain and, when necessary, protect and restore the integrity of the system.

Most of contemporary Western biomedicine is guided by the belief that the body is a machine whose function is production and reproduction. Disease and injury are seen as the result of malfunctioning parts that will respond to manipulation, suppression, stimulation, replacement, or removal. Diagnosis is based on a taxonomy of symptoms, with little attention to their origin, and clusters of similar symptoms are treated identically.

Systems theory and complexity theory are revealing that model to be flawed and unscientific. Our bodies are not machines, but self-organizing systems that adapt to change. The elements of those systems will always work in concert to ensure survival in the best ways that the information and resources available to it indicate. There is, in essence, no such thing as a maladaptive response; there are only responses based on faulty perception or wrong information, and often the only thing that can change the system's response is a change in the information the system has about the organism's experience of the world. (Unless there is significant organ damage.)

Simple things are easy for science to understand, explain, and predict. If you drop a ball, gravity will pull it toward the center of the earth, causing it to fall. Other factors do come into play—the speed and direction of the wind, the height and angle from which you drop the ball—but they are easy to factor in. You can come up with an equation that will reliably predict when and where the ball will hit the ground.

When we begin to look at more complex phenomena, like weather, simple models don't work as well to explain what is happening. This is why a weather forecast is likely to be less accurate than predictions about dropped balls.

Edward Lorenz, who worked on early computer models of the atmosphere, discovered that exceedingly small changes in one part of a system could create big changes in another part of the system. He would become famous for making the analogy that a butterfly flapping its wings in one part of the world could create—or prevent—a tornado in a distant part of the planet. Describing such events is one thing, predicting them is another, made complicated by the fact that every element of a large, complex system has its own complex and ever-changing behaviors and is made up of nesting systems with their own complexity. The way the temperature and currents of the water of a lake change the weather is a smaller version of the ways in which the temperature and currents of an ocean do, and both are microcosms in liquid form of the great ocean of air that is the earth's atmosphere.

If we see the mathematics and physics of our dominant culture as having their roots in the rationalist natural philosophy of Classical Athens, then we can say that it took "Western" science millennia to begin to grasp these complexities. Indigenous science, working with embodied intuition and with knowledge that arises from direct connection to the wind and rain and snow and sun and the living world around us, has always had more nuanced and accurate ways of predicting and describing changes in weather than conventional meteorology has.

The same is true of our bodies. We can see the conditions within our body as our internal weather, and—like changes in the planet's weather—changes in our body can never be entirely understood or described in linear ways. The longer a condition endures, the truer this becomes.

Let's look at hypertension, for example. The body elevates its blood pressure because it perceives the world as in some way unsafe, and it wants to be ready to respond to those threats. So a physician or an herbalist intervenes by giving, say, hydrochlorothiazide or Dandelion *(Taraxacum officinale)* to increase urination, reducing the volume of fluids in the body and thus reducing blood pressure. That works for a while, but the body still realizes the world still is not safe, so it increases angiotensin levels in response in order to increase arterial tension—and then the physician gives an angiotensin-converting enzyme (ACE) inhibitor, and the herbalist responds with Reishi *(Ganoderma lucidum)*. The body makes an end run around the process by increasing levels of norepinephrine, the physician gives a beta-blocker to shut down the beta receptor sites for norepinephrine, and the herbalist gives an adaptogen. Whatever response the practitioner brings, the body keeps finding new ways to elevate the blood pressure, because elevating blood pressure is an adaptive response to living under constant threat.

Any of these strategies can play a necessary role in temporarily lowering blood pressure to prevent heart attack or stroke. But none of them will be effective in the long haul. The only thing that will make a permanent change in blood pressure is a shift in your experience that makes the world feel safer and/or an increase in confidence that assures you that you can deal with it. Until the information that is informing the system's actions changes, the system will continue to find ways to respond to the existing information.

From the Qi of Chinese medicine and the Prana of Ayurveda to the Vital Force of nineteenth-century Physiomedicalist herbalism, people around the world and throughout history have spoken of a force that moves coherently through the body, giving life to its organs and tissues. When it flows properly, we experience health. When its flow is blocked or reduced—or when it burns too hot and fast—we experience disease.

Working in the first half of the twentieth century, psychologist and biophysicist Wilhelm Reich observed this moving, pulsing energy at work in human bodies—and in the simplest life forms. He called it *orgone* and noted that its motion—its expression—was guided by sensory information. "Living nature, in contrast to the nonliving, responds to stimuli with 'movement' or 'motion' = 'emotion.' It necessarily follows, from the functional identity of emotion and plasmatic movement, that even the most primitive flakes of protoplasm have sensations. The sensations can be understood directly from the responses to stimuli. These responses of plasmatic flakes do not differ in any way from those of highly developed organisms. There are no lines to be drawn here" (Reich 1973).

Today we know that slime molds can learn and alter their behavior according to sensory stimuli, and that complex signals sent between plants along mycelial networks result in plants receiving new information and altering their chemistry. We, too, respond to sensory information. Part of that sensory information is the set of electromagnetic fluctuations detected by neurons in the heart that the amygdala and the right frontal cortex of the brain interpret as emotion (for more on this, see Buhner 2004).

Reich noted that tension in the muscles and fascia blocks the flow of orgone through the body, resulting in changed behaviors at the level of tissue, organ, organism, and consciousness. Rigidity restricts motion. Motion defines life. The invitation back into motion comes through eliciting changes in sensation.

He observed particles of orgone that he called *bions*. Most of Reich's scientific colleagues rejected his theories and findings on ideological grounds, without investigating them themselves. However, contemporary biophysicists' description of biophotons, weak photons emitted from the DNA at the nucleus of a cell, bear an uncanny similarity to Reich's description of the bions he saw in his microscope in both living and decaying tissues.

Our life and our bodies are not apart from the rest of the living universe. Reich observed and worked with orgone in our atmosphere, and he perceived it as animating stars and galaxies. To put it in more expressly animist terms than Reich himself used, the forms of stars and clouds and people and animals and plants are particular arrangements that matter and energy take on for the purpose of experiencing the universe. Animist herbalism seeks to remove obstacles to the flow of life through us and to nourish that flow until the matter and energy contained within us yearn for dissolution.

Every response of a cell, a tissue, an organ, an organism, or a community— be it a physiological or behavioral response—is the system's best attempt to meet its needs with the resources and information available. The task of the healer is to understand what the system is responding to and why it is responding the way it is responding. If we seek to change the response, we need to change the information driving the response or give the system another way to accomplish what it needs to accomplish. That change in information needs to be a change in sensory information.

4. Humans need connection with other humans and with other-than-human beings to maintain optimal health.

Our ancestors evolved in a world that they experienced as alive and connected to them, speaking to them in many ways. Their bodies were attuned to the rhythms of wind and water, the sound of the air moving beneath an Eagle's wing, the exhalations of Cedar and Honeysuckle and Datura, the scents in the air, and with the pheromones of desire in each other's heartbeats.

Our biology is much the same as theirs, but our lives today are full of threats and assaults and noise that we cannot make sense of. When we experience things that overwhelm our senses, and when we experience situations in which we cannot imagine a positive or even acceptable outcome, we become disconnected from ourselves—our cognitive capacities decline and then shut down, our sense of what is happening within our bodies and in the world around us becomes narrowed to our perception of the most immediate threat in our world, and we prepare to deal with that threat, alone, by fighting, fleeing, or freezing. Our immune responses become dysregulated, as the body releases inflammatory compounds intended to deal with any injury that might result from the threat. Our digestion goes off-line. Our heart beats too quickly or too slowly and gets stuck in that response. Our blood sugar and blood pressure spike.

We come back into regulation by coming back into connection with our own bodies and our own web of relations. Most forms of psychotherapy seek to bring us into regulation by helping us come into healthy relationship with other humans—but human relationships are not the only relationships that can be therapeutic.

Connecting with plants, animals, and fungi can help to draw us back into embodied presence—especially if our history of human interactions is fraught with pain, fear, and struggle. We have an immediate, visceral set of responses to the presence of plants. When we breathe in their scents, our smooth muscles relax, we become more sensitive to hormonal signals inside and around us, and our nervous systems move into a state of coherence that recalibrates the function of our internal organs. As Guido Masé writes, "aromatics bring us into focused, flowing balance and help us function more efficiently" (2013). We seek the shade of trees in summer, and the kiss of blades of grass glazed with dew.

They are our kindred. They bring us profound medicine. And that kinship is part of the medicine.

5. Plants and fungi are not inert materials for the production of medicine, they are living beings with their own intelligences, so I seek to be in reciprocal relationship with the plants and fungi whose help I engage in healing.

This reciprocal relationship includes supporting the health of wild populations of our medicine beings and the ecologies that give rise to them.

I tend to work with very small doses of herbal and fungal medicines—one to five drops of a tincture at a time—just enough to give the body new sensory information so that fewer plants and fungi need to give their bodies and their lives to transforming human experiences. Sometimes I do not have people take herbs internally at all—instead, I may send them to visit a plant.

Out of respect for the plants and fungi that are involved in my healing work, my therapeutic goals always have an ecological dimension. I seek to help people regain their ability to perceive and act in accordance with their connection to and interdependence with the other members of the human and other-than-human communities they belong to by bringing them into states of open-hearted embodied presence. I do not seek to make it easier for people to continue to participate in an ecocidal culture. I especially do not disrespect the lives of the plants and fungi whose bodies we use as medicine by using them to enable the continuation of ways of being and thinking and seeing and feeling and unfeeling that threaten the well-being of their kin.

6. Plants and fungi belong to themselves.

While traditional relationships between plants and fungi and the Indigenous cultures that arose alongside them need to be honored as part of the ecology of a place, plant and fungal knowledge is a continuing revelation arising from all authentic and sincere relationships with the plants and fungi themselves.

For many years, I lived in a bioregion where Devil's Club grows. Coast Salish peoples have long engaged the plant in protection magic—but, though their ritual and medical science and technology inform my understanding of the plant, I do not engage it using their cultural practices. I came to know Devil's Club on its own terms and visited it regularly, bringing offerings and prayers, and harvesting it according to instructions the plant itself gave me.

I can tell you that Devil's Club grows where the forest has been disrupted by a clear cut, a landslide, or a flood. It protects rich soils and the wildflowers that grow in them, because its spiky stalks prevent big creatures from blundering over them, and its great leaves shade the ground. I can tell you that it is so hard to remove by hand that it stopped the northward expansion of the railroads in British Columbia. I can tell you its green buds tipped with purple pulsing life in spring.

But you still will not know Devil's Club. And Devil's Club will not be ready to join you in your work until you have made your own relationship. And then your magic and medicine will not resemble mine.

7. Beauty and wonder are ways we recognize the healthy flow of life.

Our innate aesthetic sense is rooted in the resolution into meaning of the gestalt of emotional and sensory information being processed by the right frontal cortex of the brain from the signals coming from the heart to the amygdala to the "right brain." (For more on this, the heart as an organ of perception, see Buhner 2004.) When we train ourselves to shift our aesthetic response away from the learned judgments of our talking, thinking minds and toward the responses of our hearts and our bodies as a whole, we begin to perceive beauty wherever there is healthy flow. The meaning we make creates context for memories and experiences, new and old. The structure of our brain shifts accordingly.

Our aesthetic sense is also deeply connected with our capacity to recognize patterns, especially those patterns that represent the relationship between forms and functions. The architect Louis Sullivan had the famous insight that form follows function. We see this in the way that the branching networks of information exchange between plants and fungi—the intertwining of plant rhizomes and fungal mycelia—resemble the structure of the human nervous system. The same pattern repeats when we map the distribution of galaxies in the known universe and superimpose their forms and placement onto their lines of connection—a fact with profound cosmological implications that suggest that not only is the planet alive and conscious but the universe itself may be as well.

Herbalists have long looked at the physical form of plants' bodies for clues to how they will work with human bodies, a principle known as the *doctrine of signatures.* There is a crude and easily ridiculed version of this principle that tends to be reduced to memorized sets of correspondences divorced from embodied experience. A more subtle and nuanced approach to recognizing signatures comes from meditation on the form of a plant. The heterodox Christian philosophers Paracelsus and Jakob Boehme—whose writings defined Western understandings of the doctrine in the sixteenth and seventeenth centuries—both believed, as Matthew Wood writes, that "the whole natural world corresponds to the archetypal world, which gives it form and meaning" (1998). In other words, the physical form of any life form is a reflection not only of its function but also of its essential nature, the qualities that make an Oak an Oak, a Dolphin a Dolphin, and a person a person. As living beings, we have the innate capacity to understand this language of form at an intuitive level. (Matthew Wood's own work provides beautiful examples of how a contemporary herbalist can use the doctrine of signatures to discover overlooked and novel dimensions of a plant's medicine.)

This is true at the molecular level as well—molecules with similar structures tend to have similar functions and tend to show up in parts of organisms that have similar forms and functions. For example, the human body uses the neurotransmitter serotonin to stimulate the growth of new neural connections. Plants use either serotonin or auxin, a rooting hormone with a serotonin-like molecular structure to stimulate rhizomic growth. The *Psilocybe cubensis* mushroom uses psilocybin and psilocin to stimulate mycelial growth. These compounds also stimulate root growth in the grasses *Psilocybe cubensis* grows with symbiotically, and they stimulate the formation of new synaptic connections in human brains. (Stephen Buhner goes into this eloquently and at great length in his book *Plant Intelligence and the Imaginal Realm* [2014], and I will touch on this biology again later in this book.)

Our bodies intuitively recognize this chemistry through the ways they respond to the scents and tastes of plants and the somatic shifts their constituents create in the body. Understandings of plant medicines rooted in direct, embodied experience tend to outpace those based on pharmacology by decades or even centuries.

Aesthetics are also central to good herbal formulation. A proper herbal formula will feel like a single herb to the body and will engage the senses fully.

My medicine is also a bardic medicine that begins to break down the distinction between the literal and the metaphorical. What we call the "literal" is an attempt to impose a single set of colonial metaphors on the world. What we call the "metaphorical" can be a potent tool for changing the meaning of information, sensations, and experiences by giving them new context.

The Irish god Manannán Mac Lir sees the sea as a field of wildflowers. The Zen poet Dogen saw mountains as slowly moving rivers of stone and rivers as swiftly moving mountains of water. I see all these things and more.

In my worldview, it is not mere whimsy to equate a river and a galaxy—both are alive and flowing. And so are you. And so am I. And so are we.

Together, these seven principles underlie and give rise to a system of healing that honors the intelligence and life of our bodies and of the living world from which they arise.

At its core, this approach to healing is about creating the conditions that allow for healthy flow. We can shift that flow through sensory impulses that stimulate the body to respond differently. Those sensory experiences create new synaptic connections when they are novel and reinforce existing ones when they are repeated.

Hot, spicy things stimulate the flow of blood and sensation. The aromatic scents of plants invite the opening of the senses. Bitter tastes stimulate the part of the nervous system in the gut, bringing us grounding. The acrid taste—the sensation of burning at the back of the throat—induces muscular relaxation, as do profoundly bitter tastes. The sweet taste brings a sense of nourishment.

Also, color has its purpose and meaning in plants and is taken into account consciously and subconsciously. From the aurora borealis to our electric body, does it not make sense that color gives us clues to our healing just as it gives clues to our condition? We intuitively recognize that when tissues are redder than usual, they are experiencing inflammation—we don't need the intellectual understanding of the fact that the redness arises from an increased flow of oxygenated blood into those tissues (though such an understanding does give context for the meaning we derive from seeing tissues turn red). Color is an important part of the signatures of plants as well: the deep red of Hawthorn berries, for example, evokes thoughts of blood and of heat, and Hawthorn is a profound medicine for inflammation in our blood vessels.

All of these sensations change what it feels like to inhabit a body in a particular moment, which changes the way the body responds. When we feel safe and free, movement, sensation, and blood flow freely through the body, promoting healthy organ function and the growth and repair of tissues. When we feel afraid or overwhelmed, that flow is blocked. When we feel depressed, that flow is diminished.

The most salient experiences we have create the strongest memories. The neural connections created by those memories are strengthened each time we repeat or remember those experiences. Those memories, in turn, shape the way we perceive new sensations and experiences—they shape what we notice, what we register as significant, and what meaning and context, both conscious and subconscious, that we give to events in our inner and outer worlds.

This is not to say that disease is the result of negative thinking. What I am speaking about is not a question of thought or belief, but rather a question of what it feels like to be you in the world in this moment and the way your body interprets and acts on that feeling.

For me, the distinction works best when I think about the model of the three-fold self that I learned to work with during my training as a priest of the Feri tradition, a shamanic tradition that found its modern expression on the west coast of North America in the second half of the twentieth century, through the teachings of Victor Anderson.

From an early age, Victor was mostly blind and profoundly psychically gifted. Past life memories and spirit visitations began coming to him as a child. Native, Mexican, and African healers and shamans in the communities where he grew up, in New Mexico and Oregon, recognized his gifts and worked to heal and train him, much to especially his mother's consternation. As a young adult in the 1930s, he found a coven of witches in Ashland, Oregon, who invited him to join them. Several years later he met and married Cora Ann Cremeans, who had grown up in Alabama, having her own spirit encounters and learning bits of Irish and Scots-Irish folk magic from her grandfather, who was called a druid. Others in Alabama, from kind Christians who did not frown on folk ways to mysterious people and her own paranormal experiences and dreams, helped her to recognize Victor as her soul mate. Their marriage and their shared practice, along with Victor's wide reading and profound intuition, shaped the insights, orientation, cosmology, ethics, and practices that would become known as the Feri tradition. One of their early initiates, Gwydion Pendderwen, whom Victor considered a spiritual son, brought more Irish and Welsh elements into the tradition as it developed. (For a sense of that approach and of who Victor was, see Benavidez et al. 2017.)

Victor noted that many societies throughout history have worked with three-fold models of the self. He spoke most frequently of Hawai'ian, Yoruban, and kabbalistic expressions of this concept, but he also recognized its presence in the three cauldrons, or three fires, of the Irish tradition and in the Christian Trinity. Others have pointed to analogues in Vedic and Daoist systems. For simplicity's sake, I will refer to these three selves by descriptive English names used by some of us in the tradition—the Human Self, the Animal Self, and the God Self. Matthew Wood works with a similar system derived from Hawai'ian tradition as interpreted (partially through the lens of a Judeo-Christian worldview) by the missionary and scholar Max Freedom Long.

What we call the Human Self is the part of us that operates in the realm of words, symbols, ideas, beliefs, categories, and abstractions. We can roughly understand it as having its seat in the left frontal cortex of the brain. It is what gives form to art, what drives science, what inspires technology. It is also the only aspect of the self that is validated and given voice by the dominant

22

culture. Disconnected from the rest of our being, it tends to become rigid and tyrannical. As Wilhelm Reich wrote, "The more the thought process is removed from reality, the more intolerance and cruelty are needed to guarantee its continued existence" (1973).

The Animal Self is the part of ourselves that experiences sensation and emotion. We can roughly understand it as having its seat in the neurological nexus that involves the nerves of the genitals, enteric nervous system (the "gut brain," which not only regulates digestion but also senses the electromagnetic and kinetic information moving through the fascia of the rest of the body), the neurons of the heart (which sense electromagnetic change in our inner and outer worlds), the amygdala (which filters and processes those signals along with the information coming in from the hormonal content of the blood), and the right frontal cortex of the brain (which assigns meaning to all of this). The Animal Self knows things not by what they are called or how they are categorized, but by how they feel. It thrives on pleasure and loving connection. It holds the memory of trauma and helps us avoid repeating devastating events by making us react strongly to the sensations associated with them. The stories the Human Self tells about the world evoke particular emotional responses from the Animal Self. It often experiences the judgments of our Human Self as instilling guilt, shame, and fear, which it also tries to avoid. Its experience of the world is the felt sense that governs our body's physiological responses to what is happening within and around us. Disconnected from the rest of our being, it tends to pursue pleasure and avoid pain without contextualizing them in a broader framework of experience. In connection with the world, it is capable of feeling things the Human Self cannot yet imagine and conveying to it new senses of possibility.

The God Self is the part of us that understands our own infinity. This is more than a theological concept. The more we understand our own bodies, the more we understand that we are microcosms that contain countless species acting symbiotically to support the continuation of one experience, one consciousness. In turn, these countless species are part of a larger macrocosm of human, ecological, and, ultimately, cosmic connection. There is no fixed boundary to who we are, where we begin and end. The matter and energy contained within our bodies is recycled and exchanged with the world around us over and over again and exists in dynamic relationship with the rest of the matter and the energy in the universe. This is a concept the Human Self cannot fully comprehend, but in moments of profound opening, our Animal Self experiences that reality viscerally. The sensations and emotions of the Animal Self are received by the God Self as a kind of somatic prayer.

Intervening at the level of belief and thought is intervening at the level of the Human Self and will often have little effect on the felt sense of being alive, except to the extent that shifting its judgments can sometimes partially shift emotional responses to a part of someone's inner or outer world. We change the experience of the Animal Self by changing what it feels, shifting its reality by engaging the senses, creating somatic shifts that, in turn, present the Animal Self with a new reality to map and imagine and that open the way to connection with the world beyond us, including our own infinity. Such shifts are not bounded by cultural limitations, except in so far as we experience the judgment of the Human Self. The Human Self responds to those new experiences in one of two ways: it either changes its structure of beliefs, and hence our brain structure, to accommodate the new experiences, or it changes the memory and meaning of those experiences to fit into its existing belief structure.

Working with *drop doses* of herbs, one to five drops of a tincture at a time, is one profound way of bringing these shifts. It creates the opportunity for the nervous system to send electricity across new neural pathways instead of habitual ones, especially if the person focuses their attention on the taste and scent of the herb and on the sensations it evokes in their body. Telling a true story about how and why this works, in terms accessible to the person you are helping and consistent with their world view increases the chances that the Human Self will fully integrate these new experience.

Matthew Wood introduced a generation of herbalists to the practice of *drop dosing*—a practice he learned from the writings of the Eclectic physicians of the nineteenth century.

Herbal medicines given at minute doses can instigate profound shifts in our sensory and emotional experiences. Indeed, to some extent, small "energetic" or "spirit" doses of herbs are most effective at instigating such shifts, because, with a few exceptions, they tend to be below the threshold of pharmacological activity and hence do not bring direct stimulation or sedation of particular organ functions. If you have felt a drop of Rose tincture soften and open your heart—and perhaps bring on tears—then you have experienced this phenomenon.

Our nervous and endocrine systems evolved responding to minute phytochemical inputs in the air our ancestors breathed, the water they drank, the brush of leaf and petal against their skin. We can replicate those exposures with drop doses of tinctures (as well as with having people spend time in the presence of aromatic herbs). The very fact that we innately recognize that these are the chemical and electromagnetic touch of other life forms, wild kindred, increases the salience of those experiences. When we cannot bring people to the forest, we can bring something of the forest to them.

I begin my work with people by exploring, in as much specific detail as possible, what they are feeling in their bodies. Tongue, pulse, and facial diagnosis; observation of their body language; and intuition round out my understanding. But I focus on teasing out detailed descriptions of sensation in order to help people gain an increased awareness of what is happening in their bodies and to help them recognize the first signs of the patterns they want to shift. Maybe the clenching of their abdominal muscles comes before they are conscious of their discomfort with a situation that is escalating into conflict. Maybe their ears feel hot before they know they are having an asthma attack. These levels of increased awareness give people opportunities to begin to see the moments when a shift in sensation can change the course of events.

Based on what we find through that exploration, I begin to test drop doses of tinctures with the person. I work only with herbs that I have had in my own body enough times to have a felt sense of their actions and their motion. This allows several things to take place.

First, people become full participants in the process of formulation—which can, in and of itself, be deeply healing for people who have experienced health care as something performed on them by practitioners working with dubious definitions of consent.

Second, unexpected adverse effects can be observed and treated with an antidote. These effects also give more information about what is happening in a person's body, allowing me to correct my sense of the person's experience.

Finally, people make visceral connections with herbs, which gives them a sense of what to expect from each herb, shaping their intention when they take the medicine, allowing the positive dimensions of the placebo effect to become an additive part of the medicine, amplifying the shifts the herbs themselves bring. Naturopathic physician Mitch Stargrove speaks of the placebo response as the vital force in disguise.

The shifts one herb brings point to possibilities of other herbs, and a formula emerges organically. I test the formula as a whole as well, so we can see if the herbs are playing together harmoniously and feel for any missing elements in the formula.

With enough practice in subtle attunement to the felt sense of the presences of plants and people, practitioners can extrapolate this system into one that can work over distance, through a video or phone call. This approach was shaped by watching Margi Flint and Matthew Wood in practice and adapting some of their strategies to suit my own inclinations.

The most common objection that I hear to this approach is that it will only work with people used to paying attention to the subtle shifts herbs bring. But I have seen it work with a seven-year-old child, a twenty-year-old waiter, an eighty-year-old retired banker, and a whole host of people in between. People will sometimes need encouragement and coaxing with the first herb, but once they realize that their experiences are relevant and make sense and line up with what we know about the herb, they relax into it.

By crafting each formula to shift a sensation in a particular way, I help give people tools to shift their experience. (I think of Aleister Crowley's oft-quoted statement: "Magick is the art and science of creating change in conformity with Will.") Generally, people find themselves recognizing early signs of the kinds of situations they are wanting to shift earlier and earlier, and they feel the herbs become more effective as a result—until they have resolved that particular pattern and are done with the formula.

For people with cyclical or alternating symptoms, like bipolar people or people with Hashimoto's thyroiditis, I will often give separate formulae for each set of experiences they want help navigating and encourage them to approach their conditions not as pathological, but as shifting tides that they can ride for particular purposes. I worked with a bipolar artist, for example, who used up phases to create new work and down phases to engage in introspection and contemplation. She would take one formula to help her remain grounded and centered while riding a creative wave and another to help her hold on to the spark of presence when she was in a place of inwardness and stillness. Rather than suppressing the symptoms, we worked together to find a way to allow her to be present with the flow of her life, her perceptions, and her neurochemistry.

Focusing on shifting the way a person experiences embodiment in the world returns herbal practice to working with the body's own intelligence to bring about healing.

What Does This Kind of Healing Look Like?

Conventional medicine tends to measure outcomes in terms of the absence of symptoms that mark deviation from an imagined norm, which tends to be determined by mechanistic concepts like performance and function. These concepts raise a couple questions: What is the role we are performing by living human lives? What is the function of a human being?

In some ways, military medicine is the most honest and transparent form of medicine in our culture in this regard, albeit in a horrific way. The job of a combat medic is not to help a person heal but to return troops to battle as quickly as possible. In the same way, in a culture that tends to measure the performance and functionality of people according to their ability to engage in economic production—and in which most need to be economically productive—there tends to be a focus on returning people to work as quickly as possible, without regard to understanding the conditions that gave rise to injury or disease or understanding the particular person who is being helped. There also tends to be a marginalization of people whose skills are not as easily commodified. And there is generally an assumption that there is one right and proper way to be human.

If, instead (as many cultures have throughout history, and a handful still do), we perceive the purpose of a human being to be perceiving beauty, participating in the dance of creation, or weaving and experiencing connection with the living world, then a different way of viewing humans and a different form of medicine emerge. There is no longer one right way of being human. Neurodiversity (which Nick Walker defines as "the diversity of human brains and minds—the infinite variation in neurocognitive functioning within our species" [2014b]) becomes one of the measures of a healthy community in the same way that biodiversity is a measure of a healthy forest. The goal of medicine becomes to help each person flourish in the fullness of who they are.

How Do We Gauge and Direct Such Medicine?

One way is through our innate, visceral, intuitive perception of where vitality is absent or present. Think of someone you love—the warm glow that person has when they are feeling happy and alive, the pallor they have when they are sick and depleted, the agitation they have when they are upset—all things you perceive without having to ask them anything. If the goal of our work is to support the flow of the vital force as it helps the person flower forth in the fullness of who they are, then the measure of our success is in the nature of their flowering.

In a particular moment, though, while it might be easy to assess the absence of vitality, it can be more difficult to determine the nature of the disruption a person is experiencing and the direction in which we want to nudge them.

In most traditional systems of medicine, the assessment of the nature of a disruption is identified by looking at a set of qualities our senses can easily assess: Is the person too hot or too cold? Too damp or too dry? Too tense or too lax? Don't overthink these terms—they are as simple and intuitive as they first sound.

Based on a visceral, intuitive assessment of these qualities of being, I develop a sense of how sensation, awareness, and blood flow are moving in a person's body and determine what change is required in that flow and what herbs will encourage that change.

What does this look like in practice? I view consultations as a fluid, shared exploration of what it feels like for a person to be embodied in the world in this moment. It is an attempt to provisionally answer what the late, great Dr. Oliver Sacks identified as the only two relevant clinical questions—"Who are you?" and "How do you be?" (Weschler 2015)—and to shift that way of being into deeper alignment with that sense of who that person is and who that person is becoming.

The consultation begins in the moment when the person I am working with first walks through the door. I notice their gait and their posture: How is this person literally walking through the world? What feeling arises in me in response to their bearing? What would I feel if I were holding and moving my body in that same way?

When the person and I and first look in each other's eyes, I tap into another layer of awareness. Being Autistic and knowing that human eye contact varies widely according to our neurobiology, I tend to put less stock in the question of whether or not the person makes and sustains eye contact than many other practitioners do. But I do hold to the Chinese belief that the quality of the *shen*, the essence of our consciousness and emotions, can be determined from the quality of the light in the eyes. Dull, flat eyes tend to reveal a deficiency in the core fire of the person's being. Eyes that seem to shine brightly reveal great vitality. Subtler qualities become apparent with attention and practice. The deepest tranquil bliss is to be found that eyes that seem to shine with the light of sunlight filtering through trees in summer.

It makes me think of Stephen Buhner's description of people who have the luminosity of an old growth forest.

The initial impression I get comes entirely from the way my Animal Self experiences the presence of their Animal Self. Sensory, intuitive, emotional. I begin to get a felt sense of that particular person's presence that will guide my work.

I begin our conversation by asking what the person wants to shift in their life. For some people, it will be a general sense of loneliness or disconnection. For others, it will revolve around overcoming a specific form of pain or marginalization. Some will frame the issue they want to address in psychiatric terms—depression, anxiety, post-traumatic stress disorder, insomnia. However the issue is first presented to me, I try to move our discussion out of the realm of the general and abstract and into the realm of particular embodied feelings.

I usually begin by asking them to remember a recent time when they were feeling the issue acutely up and recall how it felt in their body. If a person were, for example, having overwhelming fear arising while they are at work, I might ask them to describe what happened the last time they felt panicked. They might answer that their heart was racing and their stomach felt upset. From there I would try to elicit further detail: Did their stomach feel irritated, did it feel tense, or was there a sinking feeling? Did their body feel hotter or colder as the panic increased? Did they find themselves wanting to scream or run or hide? Did particular parts of their body feel tense or numb?

As they answer, I observe shifts in their gaze, their posture, their breath. I notice and ask them to notice where they are holding tension in their body as we talk.

We continue exploring the particulars of the sensations. How often do they feel this way? What makes the feeling better or worse? What makes it come on more or less frequently? What is usually the first sign that the feeling is coming on?

Through language, we are engaging the Human Self's capacity to organize and categorize information and create stories. But then, shifting awareness back to the experience of the Animal Self's sensory and emotional memories of the situation, we bring the focus back to the body, back to what it feels like to be that person present in the moment. We are simultaneously gathering information and honing the person's capacity to pay attention to subtler and subtler aspects of sensation and emotion.

As we talk, other issues will often come up. We investigate the ways they are connected with the primary issue the person identified.

While I am engaging the person, in the back of my mind I am beginning to notice the qualities of the particular way of being we are paying attention to. Is there an acceleration of movement, speech, and thought or a slowing down? A building intensity or a waning presence? An outpouring of expression and emotion or a turning inward or a restraint? The significance of all of these qualities will become clear in the chapters that follow, as we explore how each of the six tissue states is expressed mentally, emotionally, and physically. I am assessing where there is heat, where there is cold, where there is tension, where there is laxity, where there is dryness, and where there is stagnation.

As my sense of what is happening for the person coalesces, I outline what I think I see going on and make sure it makes sense to the person I am working with. I have permission to work to shift only the patterns that we both recognize are present. I can try to make another pattern, another layer, another dimension apparent to the person I am working with, but if they do not agree that particular pattern or aspect is present, then I do not have consent to address it.

Once we have reached agreement on what it is that we want to shift, I ask the person to remember a time when they felt safe and happy and present and viscerally alive. We go into the same depth of detail in discovering the particular sensations associated with that feeling of joyful embodiment. This gives us both a sense of what direction we are trying to move in. Ideally, the herbs I send the person home with will help to shift them from the felt sense they are trying to move away from and toward the kind of clear, strong presence that allows for the experience of embodied connection and embodied joy.

With the nature of the situation and of the direction we want to move in made clear, I begin testing herbs with the person to find the right remedies for them. My process of choosing herbs is often largely intuitive, based on my own body's memory of the felt sense of different plants and fungi. I never give someone an herb that I have not experienced extensively in my own body before.

But it is possible to describe the considerations that go into choosing an herb in somewhat rational and systematic terms. First I identify the organ or system where the person seems to be feeling the most acute manifestations of the problem. Then I think about the quality of the feeling in that part of the body: hot or cold, wet or dry, tense or lax. These two questions give me most of what I need to know. For example, I might be looking for herbs that are warming and relaxing to the digestive tract. In that case, I would be likely to want to try Chamomile, Catnip, Angelica, and Calamus.

I could just go ahead and test those four herbs with the person without refining my choice further. But often there will be specific indications, particular symptom patterns that suggest one herb over another. In this case, Chamomile would be indicated for someone who was sighing and complaining, Catnip for someone who fell silent and became withdrawn, Angelica for someone who was feeling frail and hopeless, and Calamus for someone whose mind felt cloudy when their stomach felt bloated—especially if that person also sometimes had trouble with verbal communication. (Matthew Wood's two-volume *Earthwise Herbal* [2008, 2009] is a great source for in-depth portraits of plants that provide a sense of each plant's "personality" and specific indications for each plant he describes.)

I test herbs one at a time by putting a single drop of a tincture on a person's hand and having them lick it off. And then I ask the person to become still and quiet and observe their subtle shifts in emotion and sensation. I am often amazed at the level of detail people with no previous experience of working with herbs are able to share about their experience of a single drop of a tincture. "I felt like someone was holding me and gently rocking me." "Everything got brighter, and my thoughts got clearer." "The center of my chest opened up, and I was finally able to take a deep breath."

Sometimes people need a little coaxing and encouragement. They will often think that the first thing they feel is too silly or irrelevant or completely imaginary. But some of the most beautiful and precise descriptions of the action of an herb that I have heard anyone give have been prefaced by phrases like "I didn't feel much, except ..." or "I might be making this all up, but ..." When I tell them that the experience that they think is too small to be of any importance or too farfetched to be true is actually a perfect description of a well-known action of the herb, which it almost invariably is, they become more confident.

All the while, I am also watching their body's response to the herb. Sometimes someone will respond to an herb in a seemingly paradoxical way: Chamomile might make them whinier, or Calamus might make their brain foggier. I take this as an indication that the body is not yet ready to shift the pattern in question to the degree that that herb will. Sometimes I will go for a gentler herb, sometimes I will try to test the herb together with another remedy that might soften it, and sometimes I will shift to an entirely different angle or approach. I always discuss this dynamic with the person who is having that experience.

When you are first starting to work with this method, I recommend sending the person you are working with home with a single herb to take at drop doses when they need to access the feeling it brings.

As you gain knowledge and experience, you can begin to move toward working with formulae. I suggest moving slowly in this realm, working first with pairs of herbs, and then with three-herb formulae, and only then moving on to more complex formulation.

A good formula should be geared toward bringing one shift in a person's experience. If you cannot describe what a formula is doing in a single, simple sentence or phrase, then the formula is trying to do too much. A good formula should also feel like a single herb to the person who is taking it.

Most formulae have one core herb that is addressing the main issue. This is usually the herb that you might send the person home with as a single herb, if you were not making a formula. The rest of the herbs are serving to modify or mitigate effects of that core herb. For example, if Angelica is bringing back a person's appetite and kindling a degree of hope they have not felt for a long time but is also making their heart race, I might pair it with Motherwort or Lemon Balm to calm the palpitations. Relaxing herbs like Lobelia can help release tension to allow other herbs to enter parts of the body that have been cut off from circulation and awareness. Heating herbs like Black Pepper and Ginger can increase circulation, carrying a formula further through the body.

Herbs don't always work together in formula in quite the ways we expect them to, even if we have tested each of the herbs individually, so I like to test the formula as a whole.

I typically have a person take three to five drops of their formula (or their single herb) as needed. Having a person take their remedy when the need arises rather than telling them how frequently to take it encourages them to pay deeper attention to their emotions and sensations, and that deepening of awareness is a fundamental part of the healing process. I usually have the person keep taking the formula until they no longer feel the need for it. When they reach that point, we have arrived at another layer of the onion, and it is time to begin the process over again to identify and address the new level of issues at hand.

A brief illustration: Rachel (not her real name) is in her early fifties. She is a naturally introverted person who experienced a series of traumatic events that led to her feeling profoundly alone and afraid. When she first arrived in my clinic in January, her eyes were dull, her body was shaking, and her voice was timid and tremulous. Over the previous decade, she had been on seven different antidepressants and two benzodiazepines. With medical supervision she had weaned off the antidepressants and was reducing her dosage of both benzodiazepines, but she was still feeling severe brain fog and expressed a struggle to find her voice. She experienced shallow, tight breathing with anxiety. She was physically frail and reported that small stresses and frustrations would cause big setbacks. When asked what qualities she wished to cultivate she replied that she longed for experiences of kindness, compassion, understanding, and tenderness. From the perspective of the six tissue states, she showed signs of constriction and depression, so I decided to test herbs that were warming and relaxing.

I tested Pasque Flower *(Anemone pulsatilla)* with her first state and found that it brought down her shaking. Next I gave her Borage *(Borago officinalis)*, which brought a feeling of deep, nurturing support. Both plants have bluish flowers covered in downy hairs. Together, they became a warm blanket wrapped around her. Angelica *(Angelica archangelica)* was the first herb to bring a smile to her face, and she experienced a deeper breath. The tightness and heaviness in her chest further released with Black Cohosh *(Cimicifuga racemosa)*, which brought tears of relief and release. And Calamus *(Acorus calamus)* cleared the fog in her head and brought clearer articulation. Her formula coming out of that session was:

- Borage: 60 ml
- Angelica: 15 ml
- Black Cohosh: 10 ml
- Calamus: 10 ml
- Anemone: 5 ml

The dosage was five drops as needed. I also advised strong Kava tea before bed to ease the rebound insomnia from the benzodiazepine reduction.

When Rachel came for her follow-up in early March, I walked past her in the waiting room initially, because she did not, at first glance, seem like the same person. It was as though she were the happier, calmer cousin of the woman I had seen before. Her eyes were bright, the shaking was gone, and her posture and gait reflected a greater confidence.

Against my advice and the advice of her doctor, she had stopped both benzodiazepines abruptly (which can be extremely dangerous). After a few days of insomnia and anxiety, she felt better, and then developed itchiness and profuse mucus.

She took the formula throughout the process and reported that her head felt clear, her heart felt open, her senses felt heightened, her breath was deeper, and she felt enormous gratitude. She was finding great joy in connecting with the animals living on her land.

She was still experiencing some anxiety, but the symptoms had shifted. Rather than shakiness and shallow breath, she was experiencing agitation and heart palpitations. Now she was primarily exhibiting the excited state, so I primarily tested cooling herbs.

When I tested Reishi *(Ganoderma lucidum)* with her, she felt a deep, grounded peace. With Damiana *(Turnera diffusa)*, she felt brightness and pleasure. With Wild Cherry *(Prunus serotina)*, she felt her heart rate become more even. And with Cleavers *(Galium aparine)*, she felt a cool, fluid release. Her formula coming out of that session was:

- Reishi: 30 ml

- Damiana: 20 ml

- Prunus: 20 ml

- Galium: 20 ml

  Dosage: five drops two to three times a day

While Damiana is a warming herb, its stimulating properties were balanced out by the cooling nature of the rest of the herbs in the formula.

Her last visit to my clinic was that May. This time, she was exuberant, and her hair was dyed blue. She was feeling happy to be alive and was planning her first travel in over a decade. She was seeking support in continuing the process of opening her heart. The focus now was on relieving the constricted tissue state with relaxing herbs.

Sheng di Huang (unprepared *Rehmannia glutinosa* root), used in Chinese medicine to clear excess heat from the blood, made her heart feel held. Hawthorn flower (*Crataegus* spp.) relaxed tension in her chest. Corydalis

(Corydalis yanhusuo) brought a fluid feeling throughout her body. Damiana *(Turnera diffusa)* brought a warm joy throughout her body. Pasque Flower *(Anemone pulsatilla)* brought calm. The final formula (which she refilled in August and November) was:

- Sheng di Huang: 10 ml
- Hawthorn flower: 10 ml
- Corydalis: 10 ml
- Damiana: 15 ml
- Pasque Flower: 5 ml

  Dosage: five drops as needed

When I saw her again the following spring, she was happy and well— and bringing a friend in to see me, in the hope that I could help him emerge from a profound depression.

Having looked at the practical and the particular, let us broaden our view now to look at how our lives intertwine with the life of the world and how an animist herbalism can understand, contextualize, and shift our experiences and the ways we engage the life within and around us. These patterns will inform the ways in which we engage herbs as allies in healing and transformation. The approach I lay out here is my own, blended together from elements of herbal and magical tradition, ancestral stories, and modern science in ways that would seem heretical to those devoted to centering and relying primarily on any one of these ways of knowing.

My friend and mentor Margi Flint calls her approach "mongrel herbalism," because it blends elements of many systems and traditions favoring what works and proves true in practice.

I liken my own approach to the fruit of the Crab Apple. Writing of the Crab Apple, Henry David Thoreau, who loved the Maine woods where I live, wrote: "Our wild apple is wild only like myself, perchance, who belong not to the aboriginal race here, but have strayed into the woods from cultivated stock."

The ancestors of the Crab Apple trees that grow here were brought from Europe and shaped and tended by human hands and human intention to try to produce a uniformly sweet fruit. Over time, some orchards were left untended, and some seeds were spread to wilder places by Bears and Deer and Waxwings and Cardinals and Buntings and Wrens. Combining their ancestral memory of European forests with their lived experience of the soil and wind and rain and snow of a very different time and place, they changed. They grew tart fruit that tasted more like the fruit the first people to gather Apples would have known—but also new and different in subtle ways even from the other Crab Apples that grew across the ridge or on the other side of the river.

I am neither of the culture around me nor of the culture of my ancestors. What I write here might be less strange to my ancestors than it would be to my neighbors, but it would be new and different to both.

Come, taste of this feral fruit and the wild waters that nourish the tree on which it grows.

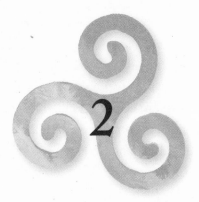

2

THE OTHERWORLD WELL

For as long as I can remember, my Da has always brought holy water from the shrine of Our Lady of Knock when visiting people in the hospital—a quiet, humble ministry that has its recent origins in rituals of the Irish Catholic diaspora, but animist roots in far older traditions of our people.

Knock is a village in County Mayo in the West of Ireland, where, on a late August evening in 1879, people coming home from gathering hay or harvesting turf in preparation for the coming winter witnessed the appearance of Mary, dressed in white robes and holding a golden Rose and attended by St. Joseph and St. John the Evangelist.

This was a generation after An Gorta Mór, the Great Hunger, brought on by the British demand that Ireland keep exporting food to its colonial masters while the potatoes the Irish people had depended on for sustenance were destroyed by late blight. Potatoes had been the principal food for the

Irish since the destruction of older food sources during the scorched-earth campaign of the British commander Oliver Cromwell two centuries earlier. It had been, in many ways, a second wave of the same genocide the people's great-grandparents had survived or perished in. During the time of hunger, people wandered from town to town searching for food, many collapsing in the streets. Others, huddled in cottages, died of diseases that spread rapidly through a traumatized and malnourished population. People called out to Mary, to Jesus, to St. Brighid, and in some places, to older spirits as well, for mercy and aid. To those who survived and to their children who grew up under occupation from the same forces that had allowed so many to die preventable deaths, Mary's apparition at Knock was an affirmation that their prayers had not gone unheard.

Our Lady of Knock played an important role in my childhood religion: among the descendants of Daniel O'Donoghue and Nora O'Meara in the heavily Irish Catholic parishes north of Boston, there was never a funeral or a memorial service where we did not sing her hymn. The hymn bore a promise that "the Lamb will conquer, and the woman who holds up the sun will shine her light on everyone."

That image of the woman holding up the sun conjures the image of far older figures than the mother of Christ: Áine, solar goddess of abundance, and Brighid of the bright flame, a goddess of healing whose name and mantle would be taken on by a Catholic saint said to be the midwife of Christ. St. Brighid is second only to Mary and Jesus in her level of veneration among the Irish and the Irish diaspora (and anyone who has spent time in an Irish Catholic house on either side of the Atlantic will know that Mary is venerated to an equal or greater degree than her son).

The name of the site of that Marian apparition, Knock, is an anglicization of the Irish Gaeilge word *cnoc*, which means "hill" or "mound." An older near synonym for *cnoc* is *sidhe*—a word that refers both to the burial mounds of Ireland's pre-Gaelic Neolithic tribes and to the beings the old gods, from whom the modern Irish people trace the oldest indigenous side of their roots, became when they vanished from the world to escape the onslaught of a civilization whose ways were too brutal for them. We can think of the font of holy water at the shrine of Our Lady of Knock as taking the older place of the well near the burial ground as a place for calling on healing from the source of all life—a connection I only really understood once I was in Ireland.

In Liscannor, just south of the Cliffs of Moher on the rocky coast of County Clare, there is a well fed by a cold, wild spring, where Brighid was honored once as a goddess and now as a saint, at the foot of a mound where new and old graves stand above the ancient tombs of chieftains and kings, buried close to the waters that could carry them into the arms of their wild lover, the land itself to which they were ritually wed at their coronations. A short way up the hill is a *clootie tree*—a tree where people tie strips of cloth as they make prayers for the health of their families and the fertility of their land.

In the first days of September, in 2017, I found myself standing by the tree, looking down toward the well, praying for the healing of the forests I had just learned were burning in the Columbia River Gorge where I then made my home. I hung one of my most prized possessions from a branch—the tip of a Deer antler on a rawhide string given to me by someone I loved when I first came to the gorge—hearing a voice echo within me saying, "a big prayer requires a big offering."

I went down to the well itself, contained now by stone walls lined with photos of the sick and the dead, Brighid's crosses woven with reeds, and candles burning in small grottoes, drank deeply of the cold, cold water, light brown with the tannins of the peat it had filtered through.

There was a steady stream of people coming, bearing photographs and rosaries, even on a weekday morning. After making their prayers, many would gaze into the water. Tradition says that if you see an image of a Salmon in the play of light and shadows on the water, the person you are praying for will be healed: echoes of a still older way of seeing the world.

There is no surviving evidence of an Irish creation story—perhaps the birth and origin of the world is not as universal a fascination as our contemporary culture assumes. But the origin of springs and rivers is another question—though as much a geographical question as a temporal one, but no less definitive of a way of being. And in Irish tradition, the waters of this world come from a single well in the Otherworld below.

John Moriarty said, "For us to learn to speak is to learn to say: 'our river has its source in an Otherworld well,' and anything we say about the hills and anything we say about the stars is a way of saying 'A Hazel grows over the Otherworld well our river has its source in' " (2006).

Within this framework, there is no distinction between physical and metaphysical geography—the dark world beneath our feet from which the wild waters come, from which the elemental essence of our being is drawn and to which it returns when we die, is not another dimension or another reality but a place, just like a hollow hill or an ocean or the surface of the moon or the cold black space between stars.

Sorcerer and folklorist Robin Artisson, whose work translates elements of the traditional Irish, Scottish, Cornish, Breton, and Welsh Fayerie Faith into the context of the spiritual ecology of contemporary North America, writes that the Unseen World "is not separate from or 'beyond' this world. It is deeply resident inside the world that we sense. It is an interior dimension to sensual things, a dimension that it just as natural as anything else we encounter with our senses" (2018).

The Unseen World is the darkness of the womb and of the grave and of the oceans from which life emerged and the emptiness from which the first matter and energy emerged. In the Irish mythos, it is the place to which the Tuath Dé, the Tribe of the Gods, the people who had brought magic and knowledge from the North and learned to work with and change the flows of wind and water, returned when they left this world, driven back by the onslaught of civilization, a world whose entry places lie in ancient burial mounds and in the places where lone Hawthorns grow. It is that dimension of being where the infinite flows into the particular. Holy places and wild places, within ourselves and in the world, are where we can most easily meet (and sometimes cross, but not without danger) that boundary.

It is also within our inner waters—in our blood and our interstitial fluids that carry chemical, kinetic, electrical, and photic signals through our bodies.

In many cultures, water has long been associated with our emotions, our dreams, and our unconscious knowings. The late neuroscientist Candace Pert famously asserted that the body is the unconscious mind and that our hormones are molecules of emotion. It is at this level of being that we viscerally understand and directly experience our relationship with all life.

In that Otherworld, the oldest creature in the world—the ancestor of all Salmon—swims in the well, eating the nuts that fall from the Hazel trees whose branches spread over the well from which the rivers flow, taking in all the wisdom the Hazel drew from the soil of that Otherworld and carrying it into our own. The Salmon of life within us is a descendant of that Salmon that knew the waters of that Otherworld. Wild water welling up from the ground brings a reminder of that world and our relation to it, and it can bring a new infusion of life or carry someone more smoothly toward death.

Wells are sacred to Brighid who presides over the bright half of the year in the old Irish calendar, from her festival of Imbolc, in early February, when Sheep giving their first milk of the year marks the loosening of winter's grip on the land until Lughnasadh, in early August, which marks the harvest of the first grains and first fruits as plants focus on sending what sunlight they can still gather into their roots and dropping their seed into the earth.

The wild waters that rise from these wells have spent hundreds of years underground, and as they make their way back to the surface, they filter through soils infused with the chemical traces of roots and leaves and flowers and fruit that dissolved back into the earth when they died. In places where the water filters through peat, they carry the aromatic molecules of forests and fields that existed thousands of years ago. These wild waters are medicine from the time of our ancestors, carrying the memory of a different world.

Water, by its very nature, is fluid, malleable, and receptive. As a universal solvent, it tends to dissolve the boundaries between things. Moriarty wrote that it was at the Otherworld Well that he "learned that being human was a habit that could be broken" (2009). By going to the wellspring of all life, it becomes possible to remember our connection with all things.

When our tissues dry out, they become rigid, and that rigidity in our tissues leads to rigidity in our response to the world. We restore their pliability with herbs whose polysaccharides, which make them mucilaginous, are similar in structure to those that make up the fluids in our own bodies that lubricate our fascia, coat and protect the linings of our respiratory and genital and urinary and digestive tracts, carry electrons and hormones through the spaces between our cells, and form our cell membranes. Mullein, Solomon's Seal, and Shatavari have particular affinities for the synovial fluid that lubricates our joints and connective tissues, so they are the demulcent herbs that play the greatest role in my practice. Drop doses of these medicines can encourage the secretion of new fluid, larger doses of Solomon's Seal and Shatavari are more materially restorative.

Fats are essential as well—among other things, we use them to manufacture our hormones and neurotransmitters, to give structure to neurons, and to create the cholesterol rafts that float on the polysaccharide oceans of our cell membranes that are central to cell signaling. Without adequate fats, our relationship with the world becomes a dry and brittle one, we are unable to fluidly respond to our experiences, and thus we either become stuck in hyper-reactivity or unable to mount a response to the world at all.

A misunderstanding of the nature and role of dietary fats has made low-fat diets and cholesterol-reducing medications ubiquitous. The lack of dietary fats and the disruption of cholesterol metabolism by statin drugs leads to problems with neurological signaling and inadequate hormone and neurotransmitter production, leaving the nervous system energetically depleted and brittle, and leading to cognitive decline and possibly even to the disruption of intercellular communication.

Questions have arisen about whether there is any benefit to reducing the quantity rather than improving the quality of dietary fats at all. Heat-damaged unsaturated fats and the trans fats they become do elevate inflammation, and trans fats may create structural problems at the cellular level. However, the formation of the type of cholesterol implicated in forming arterial plaques, very low density lipoprotein, is linked not to high fat consumption but to high sugar consumption, and there is also some evidence that its presence may be a symptom rather than a cause of cardiovascular damage, with lipid plaques in the body generally serving to protect damaged tissues, and the plaques in this instance covering lesions in the blood vessels caused by chronic inflammation and possibly by the excess sugars themselves and the resulting excess insulin.

I personally favor high-quality animal fats for my clients and in my own diet. They are the most structurally similar to the fats in our own bodies. Because fat is, like water, a medium that dissolves and carries other substances, it is important to make sure the fats come from animals that have had minimal exposure to environmental toxins. Also, both for ethical reasons and because adipose tissues also contain residues of the hormones moving through an animal body, it is important to make sure those animals have lived healthy lives. Animals that have been allowed to eat their natural diet—wild fish and game, grass-fed Sheep and Cattle, Chickens allowed to peck about and eat bugs, woodlot-fed Pigs—will have higher levels of anti-inflammatory omega-3 fatty acids in their diets and lower levels of pro-inflammatory omega-6 fatty acids in their tissues. For those who don't eat foods that come from the bodies of animals, I favor Avocado and Coconut oils because of their molecular stability—saturated fats are solid at room temperature because their molecular structure renders them compact and non-reactive, and because of this they are not prone to oxidation or to structural damage in the same way that unsaturated fats are, because of unoccupied binding sites within their molecules that want to bond to oxygen atoms. Unsaturated fats damaged by heat and oxidation increase inflammation within our bodies, which then inflames the senses and the mind.

I was a vegetarian myself for many years, but when I began engaging more deeply with plants and fungi and their consciousness I was no longer able to draw a clear ethical line for myself between the taking of life from different biological kingdoms. Industrial agriculture, both industrial meat production and industrial cultivation of grains and legumes, has horrific ecological and health consequences across the board, and it disconnects us from the food we eat and the ecological communities we share with the plants and animals whose lives we take to sustain our own. Breaking away from these monolithic systems requires making way for a diversity of local food systems and a diversity of diets, and we each need to navigate the ethical, economic, ecological, and health questions involved in ways that make sense in our own particular context. I am always willing to engage in conversation about these questions and always loathe to try to answer them for other people.

Before leaving the subject of fat altogether, I want to speak about the fact that our own body fat is an essential organ of our consciousness. Anatomist and philosopher Gil Hedley writes, "The living adipose is basically liquid energy and raw power suspended in a web of piezoelectrically conductive collagen fibers. Through it are transmitted fields of information from our external environment to the depths of our bodies at all times. The adipose layer is replete with specialized smooth muscle cells, whereby the tissue tone is maintained and adjusted. It is as if our soft coating of fat is a living antenna of the most sensitive kind, receiving from without and broadcasting within the waves of information that surround us" (n.d.).

High levels of body fat production may be more linked to our experience of the world than to diet and lack of exercise alone. Under the influence of cortisol released into the blood during times of continuous stress, the body favors the release of insulin over the release of human growth hormone, which, in turn, leads us to favor the production of adipose tissues over the production and repair of muscle and other tissues. We developed this response both so that we could store energy in hard times and so we could increase our body's sensitivity to its environment. When we don't have the means or context to handle the increased sensory information coming in through our body fat, many of us tend to try to dull those sensations by increasing our consumption of sugars and starches that dull our perception— which, in turn, leads to more insulin release and more body fat production in a cycle that can be difficult to break. High insulin levels, dysregulated blood sugar, stress, and their associated inflammation all are correlated with chronic issues ranging from high blood pressure to joint pain to depression.

The correlations between high body fat and poor health likely have to do with this metabolic and endocrine disruption rather than with the presence of adipose tissue itself.

Our war against body fat can become a war against our own fluid and receptive natures. It also becomes a war against our own bodies, which makes it hard for us to cultivate embodied presence in the world. It can be a war against pleasure—the sensual pleasure of enjoying food, and the sensual pleasure of the softness of our own and each other's bodies. As such, it threatens to cut us off from what nourishes us, which, in turn, can make us crave even more of the false comfort we find in processed foods engineered to stimulate dulled senses while simultaneously dulling them further.

We are watery creatures, our awareness fed by the streams of our senses. In the tradition of my ancestors, the waters of those streams of sensation were held within the body by three cauldrons in which they were cooked down and distilled into the stuff of life.

There were forests here once
where now there is only limestone
and brush and thin soil;

the waters of the well
remember flowing
through roots of Oak and Fern

and earth that knew
the footsteps
of Deer and Fox and Hare
before the time
of the long gun
and the axe.

Macha told me
to bring my people home.

But I do not know
who my people are
and the distant forests
of home
are aflame.

So, I hang the tine
of the antler
of a Stag
from the Hawthorn
by the well

and Brighid leads me
up the hill
to the grave of
an gaiscíoch
na Poblacht

inscribed in Gaeilge
in 1922.

Beneath him
lie the bones
of chieftains
and kings
buried beneath
the mound
that the waters
might carry them
back to the arms
of their wild lover,
this land.

I hear her voice
and I am undone:
priest of a burning forest
bard of a language I've lost
King of dry bones

who will embrace
this body
when I am gone?
What river
will carry
me home?

THREE CAULDRONS

E arth, water, and fire come together in the cauldron where life begins— and as we emerge from that cauldron, our choices determine the way we mediate their interactions, shaping our lives. My Irish ancestors understood the waters of our being to be held by three cauldrons warmed by three fires within the body. Understanding the nature of those three cauldrons can guide us in cultivating health.

What we know about the three cauldrons we have gleaned from a seventh-century poem, written in Old Irish, preserved in a sixteenth-century manuscript and attributed to the Bronze Age poet Amirgen. Amirgen was the bard of the tribe of Celts who first sailed to Ireland from Galatia, taking the land from the Tuath Dé, the Tribe of the Gods, who would become the faerie people, the Daoine Sidhe, when they retreated into the dark, watery underworld. Amirgen gained sovereignty by courting the spirit of the land with poetry that spoke of his unity with all things—proclaiming that he had been a Hawk flying over cliffs, a Salmon swimming swiftly, a Stag with antlers of seven tines, a drop of dew gleaming in the sun.

"The Cauldron of Poesy" speaks of the nature and origin of poetry, which was connected with creation, destruction, and transformation in ancient Irish culture, and which he spoke of as arising from what is cooked in three cauldrons within the body: the Cauldron of Incubation, which is upright within us when we are born, the Cauldron of Motion, which starts off turned on its side but can become upright if we move in good ways in response to the joys and sorrows of life, and the Cauldron of Wisdom, which is inverted when we are born, pouring down blessings on us, but becomes upright when we attain an ecstatic state, from which we pour blessing out into the world. The Cauldron of Incubation is the birth place of the Animal Self and one place where that self flows together with the God Self; the Cauldron of Motion can be seen as the meeting place of the Animal Self and the Human Self; and the Cauldron of Wisdom is the seat of the God Self that gives inspired expression through the ways in which the Animal Self experiences infinity and union giving rise to the emotion and rhythm of poetry. My favorite modern translation of the poem was done by Erynn Rowan Laurie, a poet and scholar who has played an important role in the Celtic Reconstructionist movement—where I quote from the text here, I quote from her translation (Laurie n.d.).

The Cauldron of Incubation holds the primal essence of who we are and who we will become. Amirgen describes it as having "been taken by the Gods from the mysteries of the elemental abyss." It is the place where life begins, where watery potential is distilled into solid form. It is also the place where poetry's power to create and destroy is born—from it there "pours forth a terrifying stream of speech from the mouth." I think here of the potent energy at the root in Tantrik traditions that rises along the spine, becoming the kundalini.

Most modern commentators and practitioners locate the Cauldron of Incubation in the belly, but for me, its name, its role as the place where the waters of life first enter into and become our being, and its place as the root of our primal poetic impulse all suggest the pelvis, which, in its form, is also more similar to a cauldron. I associate it with the root chakra and the sacral plexus in Westernized understandings of Vedic models of the body and with the function of the kidneys in Chinese medicine. I experience it as white—the color of starlight and bones—and a color Celtic cultures have long associated with the Otherworld. (Robin Artisson explores this connection at length in his book *An Carow Gwyn* [2018]. He connects whiteness with the pallor of death and hence with the realm of the ancestors.)

In the pulse, I feel what is happening within the Cauldron of Incubation in the quality of the flow of blood across the third position on the wrist, the one associated with the kidneys in Chinese pulse diagnosis. And I feel the influence of events there on other organs and on the body as a whole at the third depth, the bone depth, which in Chinese pulse diagnosis tells us the material condition of the organ in question.

It is the place where formlessness moves into form, where we strike the balance between structure and flow. Herbalist Subhuti Dharmananda writes (n.d.):

First, there is essence, the intertwining of yin and yang that makes up all things. It has—this time—manifested as a human, the ultimate meeting of heaven (yang) and earth (yin). The essence, as a manifestation from earlier existence through the continuing cycle of death and rebirth, gains its new chamber, the kidney, which retains it and allows it to slowly emerge in form. From this precious chamber sprouts the skeleton, and within the spine, the spinal cord and brain, and from the brain the retina and hearing mechanism. Within the bones is the marrow which generates blood. Also from the kidney emerges the reproductive organs, so as to help assure another part of the linkage between earlier existence and later existence.

The *yang* is that which seeks expression, and the *yin* is the living substance through which it manifests. The kidney *yang* is the fire that heats the Cauldron of Incubation; the kidney *yin* is the water within the cauldron.

We do need structure as well as flow. We are rivers held in by strands of protein and just enough minerals that we can stand upright and dance. To understand the nature of that structure, we turn to Brighid's dark twin, who presides over the dark months that follow, and is known by several names across Ireland and Scotland and the islands off their coasts:

Bone Mother. Cailleach Béara. Nicnevin.

In Gaeilge traditions, she is the dark bride the land becomes at Samhain.

Here, the north wind is her breath. The mountain range that shelters the lake where my house is mirrored is her spine, running south to Georgia and north and east to Ireland and Scotland.

If Brighid is the flowing water and the bright dancing flame, the Cailleach Béara is the cold solidity of the earth that holds our ancestors' bones, the darkness of the womb and the grave.

In Wales, she is Cerridwen, whose cauldron of death and rebirth is also associated with the power to shape-shift—a power that arises from our understanding that the water and proteins and minerals and fats that become our bodies had life as other bodies as well. (In the Irish tradition, that power of understanding comes from eating the body of the Salmon of Wisdom or eating the Hazel nuts that fall into the well where the Salmon dwells and the river has its source. Laurie has uncovered interesting evidence that these may be oblique references to the sacramental use of the *Amanita muscaria* mushroom, the iconic red and white mushroom of northern European folklore. I have wondered myself, drawing more from inspiration and vision than from scholarship, if the *Psilocybe semilanceata* mushroom, the Liberty Cap mushroom, which grows in Cattle and Sheep pastures across Ireland and Britain, may have filled a similar role.)

On both sides of the North Atlantic, Samhain, the time of Cailleach Béara's coronation, is the season of the Deer hunt and the culling of the Cattle herd. Throughout the winter my ancestors nourished themselves with the meat harvested at Samhain—and they broke open the bones and cooked them in great cauldrons over fires of driftwood and peat, often with seaweed gathered from the rocky shores.

In the season when the Cailleach Béara rules, we spend long nights in the shadow, confronting what we did not face in the bright light of day.

Sometimes, in the darkness, we are stripped as bare as the Oak and the Birch in the winter. In such times, I remember the wise words shared by the doorkeeper in a North American ceremony, not unlike those of my ancestors, where we prayed all night for the rising of the sun: If you use your muscles to hold yourself up through the night, you will grow tired and sore. Instead, rest into your bones and let them support you.

In Chinese medicine, the kidney is the reservoir of our ancestral inheritance, and the mother of the bone. That ancestral essence, the *jing*, is a watery thing that calcifies into solid form as we come together in the womb and as we grow in the world. It is also the source of the sexual fluids that carry and transmit our genetic inheritance.

We are learning that bone was a complex endocrine organ that evolved to help us escape from danger. When we sense danger, our bones release osteocalcin, a hormone that initiates our stress response. It is worth noting that it does this not by directly signaling the adrenals to release cortisol and adrenaline, but by shutting down the parasympathetic function of the autonomic nervous system, letting our bodies know that it is time to stop rebuilding and repairing themselves and switch into survival mode. We come back to ourselves and each other by settling into our bones.

Recent archaeological discoveries suggest that storing Deer bones to sustain the tribe through lean times is one of the oldest human practices. A practice as old as simmering those bones and gathering to tell the stories and sing the songs that remind us who we are. Songs and stories are prayers chanted over the soup that will tell the molecules of the dissolving bones what form to take as they transmute from animal bone to human flesh.

Chinese medicine teaches that stress, worry, and struggle deplete the kidney *yin*, the primal material source of bone. Broths made from roots and animal bones are one of the oldest medicines for replenishing that essence—foods harvested in autumn that sustain us through winter. There is profound medicine in these bones themselves—their collagen and their minerals help us restore our own skeleton and the collagen of our own fascia, which gives us structure as well. Sweet-tasting roots hold the energy the plant sent down into the earth, storing that energy for the months when it would be harder to gather energy from the sun—roots that reach down to subterranean water. These roots, many of them the same polysaccharide-rich mucilaginous roots that I spoke of above, help us rebuild ourselves. Solomon's Seal and Shatavari roots are associated with replenishing the sexual fluids as well, though I personally speculate that their role as aphrodisiacs may have at least as much to do with their moistening the fascia, making us more receptive to touch and presence.

Chinese medicine traditionally uses the velvet Deer scrape from their antlers and the spring pollen of the Pine to nourish the fire at the root that moves the waters we replenish with the sweet, moistening herbs—hence their modern popularity among weightlifters, who are trying to build new tissue from the elements of life, and their reputation for increasing libido, which ultimately is just life force itself. Scots Pine was a popular herb in springtime beers in Scotland before seventeenth-century cultural shifts turned beer from a brew frequently made with aphrodisiac, stimulant, and mildly mind-altering ingredients to a sedative and libido-reducing drink made with Hops. (Stephen Buhner goes into this at length in his book *Sacred and Herbal Healing Beers* [1998].) Pungent, aromatic roots like those of Osha, Angelica, and even Ginger can also stimulate the fire that warms the Cauldron of Incubation. When the fire has all but died out, the intense heat of Wormwood can rekindle its spark. Gently warming Damiana, which brings blood flowing to the pelvis, helps to connect the Cauldron of Incubation with the Cauldron of Motion.

If the Cauldron of Incubation cannot hold onto energy, especially if there is too much urination or too much discharge of sexual fluids, then astringent herbs—the herbs that make your mouth pucker when you taste them—will be indicated. If you ask most people what quality they associate with the astringent taste, they will tell you that astringent herbs and foods are drying.

Certainly, the first sensation we usually experience when we taste something astringent is a puckering of the tissues of the mouth, followed by a decrease in salivation. The puckering, not the dry sensation itself, is the keynote here—the puckering is the result of the fibers of the skin and muscle tissues binding together more tightly, which, in turn, locks in moisture, preventing it from being lost through secretion.

Astringents separate things and give them structure by reinforcing boundaries. This is true of thoughts and emotions as well as of physical fluids—though we'll discuss the former more when we discuss the Cauldron of Warming.

Astringents are often called "tonics" in old literature, because they restore tone to tissues. This way of viewing tonification is reflected in our modern concept of "muscle tone" and "muscle definition." When muscles grow weak, their fibers grow farther apart, and they begin to sag. They become less visible and less palpable beneath the skin, and they become less able to do their work. If you want your muscles to grow stronger, you carefully injure them by overloading them, causing small tears, which, when repaired, become areas where the muscle fibers are denser and more closely bound together. As muscle tone increases, muscle "definition" increases—the muscle becomes more recognizable by sight and touch and more clearly differentiated from the tissues around them.

Unfortunately you cannot use astringent herbs as a substitute for exercise to increase muscle tone. The one thing that we do know increases resting muscle tone is strengthening the connection between each muscle and the brain through conscious focus on contracting and relaxing each muscle. However, some astringent herbs will help you keep from leaking life force, giving you more energy and stamina when you do exercise, especially when combined with herbs that light the fire at the root. Schizandra, the Ginseng cousin called Eleuthero, and Damiana are a favorite combination of mine here.

Misunderstandings of what the old texts mean when they speak of tonification have led to misunderstandings of herbs—when people read in old texts that Goldenseal is a "mucus membrane tonic," they tend to assume that means it is something you should take every day to improve general mucus membrane health. What the old texts actually mean is that Goldenseal is a mucus membrane astringent. When the mucus becomes thin and runny, Goldenseal helps check its flow.

So we can best understand astringent herbs as herbs that create boundaries against the secretion, flow, and infiltration of fluids by binding tissue fibers more closely together. Chinese medicine traditionally uses Schizandra, the five-flavor berry, to prevent the leakage of *jing*. Sumac in North America and the Middle East and Rowan in Ireland and Britain have an astringency and a tartness similar to those of Schizandra (though they lack its sweetness, bitterness, and hint of peppery heat) and can be used in similar ways to strengthen the container of the Cauldron of Incubation. All three have associations with the Stag and the hunt, suggesting stamina and focused awareness. All of the plants of the Rose family are astringent, with the plants of the *Rubus* genus—Raspberry, Blackberry, Salmonberry, Thimbleberry, and so on—with their three-leafed structures that suggest the form of the pelvic musculature, having a special affinity for this lower cauldron. Blackberry root is the most astringent of the *Rubus* medicines and is my go-to medicine whenever someone is losing fluids quickly.

Oak bark is profoundly astringent and was traditionally used to tan leather. The solidity of the Oak and its ability to draw down lightning and survive the lightning strike are deeply connected with its traditional associations with kingship in Celtic cultures—pointing to the role of king as protector but also to the role of the king as the one who draws down light and fire from the heavens to give new life to the land. Mushrooms proliferate around the Oak in the wake of a lightning strike.

Daoist medicine, which had its origins in the same time as the Vedic medicine and Tantrik science that the people who would become known as Indo-Europeans carried across a continent and an ocean to Ireland in the Neolithic, speaks of our lives being a river of destiny—what we inherit from the ancestors is the water, and the pull of the planets on those waters creates motion and flow—as does the way we move in the world. It is earth that gives us structure. It is the fires of the sun melting the snow that gives movement and force.

The Cauldron of Motion is the place where the body distills its experience of the world, of the joys and sorrows of life. It is the seat of sensation (which Wilhelm Reich described as the bridge between the ego and the outer world) that gives rise to emotion (which Reich described as the movement of the organism in response to sensation) and thus the place from which we move, speak, and act in the world.

All activity, physical and mental, requires the flow of oxygenated blood to our tissues. The Cauldron of Motion is the seat of that innate intelligence that guides this flow in response to inner and outer events. When we are in a state of health, this flow is free and rhythmic, like good poetry. It is reflected in health in a free and easy flow at the middle depth of the pulse, referred to in Chinese pulse diagnosis as the blood level, which reflects what is happening with our organs at a functional level. I experience it as red.

This corresponds in contemporary biomedicine with the concept of heart rate variability. The heart is not a mechanical pump with a single, regular, repeating, staccato rhythm, but a drum whose rhythm shifts and changes in response to our experience of the world. The best predictor of cardiac health and overall health is heart rate variability, the ability of the heart to shift fluidly from one rhythm to another, which tracks closely with the strength and clarity of the signals flowing across the vagus nerve that facilitates communication between the brain and every internal organ except the adrenal glands. The best way to restore or maintain heart rate variability is to walk mindfully in a forest, inhaling the exhalations of its plants, and with them the subtle signals contained in their release of aromatic compounds that the body recognizes as an invitation to connection.

Our perception of the world plays a role in guiding the rhythm and flow of our blood. When we feel safe, embodied, and connected, we are responsive to the world around us. The "Cauldron of Poesy" tells us that is a result of a healthy turning of the Cauldron of Motion, inspired by the true joy that comes from intimate connection with the Human, the Wild, or the Divine, or with great art, and by distilling the truths revealed by sorrow. In such a state, we are physically open, and we allow what stirs within us to be expressed freely in our movement and our communication. Fear closes us, creating constriction that can either cut off the flow altogether or lead to a building of pressure as intense forces press against strong barriers, which we will explore thoroughly in the next chapter.

Physical motion gets our blood and lymph flowing, which allows us to move through our experiences. Blood carries oxygen and hormones to our tissues, lymph carries metabolic waste out of the tissues and is moved by the pressure created on lymphatic vessels by compression (through exercise that contracts the muscles—or through massage or immersion in water).

When the circulation is deficient, we become cut off from awareness of some parts of our bodies (something exacerbated by constriction) and eventually begin to lose adequate blood flow to the brain. Hot herbs like Cayenne and Rosemary and herbs like Prickly Ash and Devil's Club that create sharp sensations on the tongue (their spines are an interesting signature here) can bring us into sudden, sharp awareness, quicken the heartbeat, and send blood flowing more forcefully and swiftly through the body, especially when combined with an herb that removes the tension constricting the flow, like Lobelia. Warming herbs like Ginger, Cinnamon, Cardamom, Basil, and Sage provide gentler support for keeping blood and awareness flowing. Yarrow has the unique and mysterious ability to, as Matthew Wood says, guide the proper flow of the blood, preventing both clotting and hemorrhaging.

Fear can cause a sudden increase in the heart rate. Often this is associated with the release of histamine—a compound people best know through its association with allergies. Histamine serves multiple functions: as an immune factor, it signals the body to increase its local inflammatory response in the tissues where it is released in order to fight off infection and repair damage; as a neurotransmitter, it serves to create and consolidate negative memories so that we will avoid being injured in the same way again and respond strongly if we feel something similar to that previous injury. It also stimulates an anxious response in the amygdala that may partially explain the strong association that is being established between high histamine levels and addiction. Histamine will generate heat and redness. The leaves and flowers of many plants of the Rose family, especially Hawthorn, Rose, and Peach, are tremendously helpful in calming the physiological and emotional hyper-reactivity that are associated with histamine releases.

Reishi mushrooms and their North American cousins of the *Ganoderma* genus have a long history of being used to calm the spirit, as well as a recent history of showing a remarkable capacity for modulating inflammatory immune responses. I have found that—over time for most people, and instantly for a few—Reishi can help bring a profound sense of stillness. Matthew Becker speaks of Reishi's capacity to "pull trauma from tissues." I experience this as a kind of metabolization of experiences and memories, analogous to the support Reishi provides for the liver's work of clearing physiological toxins and metabolic waste. There is an interesting signature present here—Reishi spreads its white mycelium through the wood of old trees, slowly breaking that wood down, bringing forth the red fruiting body of the mushroom, which releases golden spores into the wind. Wood holds the memory of the experience of the tree, as evidenced by the way we can read the history of a tree's life by looking at the rings within its trunk that mark each year of its growth, so Reishi is metabolizing the tree's experience—the same thing it does for us. The red of the fruiting body suggests the blossoming of life, the golden spores dispersed on the wind suggest the luminous wisdom of a life well lived being passed on to others. The white of the mycelium, similar in form and function to our nerves, suggests consciousness reaching into the world of things past, those things to which blood no longer flows.

Schizandra, traditionally used as a meditation aid in China, combines beautifully with Reishi to calm an agitated heart. I think of Schizandra as an astringent of consciousness, gathering scattered and wandering flows of thought and emotion back inward to the heart. You could say that it helps plug leaks in all three cauldrons.

When agitation brings sudden, intense emotion to the surface, I rely on bitter mint family plants to help draw the flow of blood and awareness down lower into the body. The bitter taste is profoundly grounding, and Mint family plants, like Rose family plants, tend to be good at calming excess heat without smothering the healthy heat of vitality. Lemon Balm is indicated when agitation brings sudden flashes of anger. Motherwort is indicated when agitation brings sudden tears. If a person shows a tendency to weep themselves into exhaustion, I will add to Motherwort's grounding bitterness the gentle cooling and subtle astringency of Rose—which will slow the tears without suppressing them.

Lack of motion—mental, physical, and emotional—can make the inner waters stagnant. We find ourselves stewing in the same neurotransmitters and hormones, ruminating on grievances and sorrows, reproducing the same emotions, which leads us to release more of the same hormones and neurotransmitters and to continue stewing on them. We also find ourselves more susceptible to outside influences, be they other people's thoughts and emotions that linger with us or actual chemical influences from an increasingly toxic world. Sometimes we need medicines and rituals of purification.

Large segments of our culture often conflate and confuse purification with purging and punishing the body—something not surprising when we consider that, whether we attend church or not, and whatever we ourselves believe, the culture of the United States and the culture of global capitalism it gives rise to are shaped by a version of Christianity that views the body and its earthly desires and pleasures as corrupt and sinful. These cultural forms are marked by the alternation of periods of gluttony with periods of severe deprivation, and periods of ignoring accumulating physical and emotional toxicity with harsh, cathartic cleanses for a body we either consciously or unconsciously view as dirty and sinful, especially in the United States, where a Puritan strain runs through the culture. New Age fixation on ascension and pure light, misunderstandings and misappropriations of Vedic and Tantrik concepts by North American Yoga enthusiasts, colonics and extreme laxatives, all are rooted in a paradigm that seeks purification through discipline and punishment even though their language and their surface concepts are different from those of the fire-and-brimstone Puritanism of the seventeenth-century Massachusetts Bay Colony. This is not what I mean when I speak of purification.

Robin Artisson gives my favorite description of what purification means in the context of an animist worldview: "Purification is never about cleaning your 'gross human self' of some kind of moral stain, nor of separating yourself from any aspect of your humanity. It's simply about removing potential powers acting on you that hinder your work."

Those influences acting on us can include the influence of neurotransmitters and hormones that were appropriate to another time and place but not to the one we are in here and now—both those that we discussed above that create heightened states of reactivity and those that move us in the opposite direction—toward grief and despair.

Orientation within time depends in part on connection with seasonal cycles. As my friend and teacher Cornelia Benavidez recently reminded me, people around the world have always come together to observe the seasonal changes in the sun, the moon, and the stars. Such times were marked by shared work of planting or harvesting or hunting, followed by feasting and celebration. They were also times of ritual and prayer, when people would tap into their own bodies' sense of the changes afoot in the world and use the momentum of the winds and the currents and the shifts in the lives of plants and animals and the land and water themselves to remember how to create the same kinds of change in their inner worlds.

Ritual resets the rhythm of the heart and the blood—this is part of why drumming, singing, and dancing are some of the oldest ritual techniques in the world. In the earliest rituals we have evidence of, people donned animal skins and moved like the animals in the world around them, reminding the Animal Self how to be an animal in the season the world was entering. Most martial arts hold versions of this ancient knowledge of using movement in precise ways to change and focus consciousness and guide action in ways that are at once swift and fluid.

The rituals that connect us with the life cycles of the other-than-human beings around us also serve to orient us to cycles of birth and death in ways that allow us to face our own mortality and shift our identification from our individual bodies to the body of the world. It is worth noting that the three therapies that seem to be most effective for treating the anxiety and depression associated with the diagnosis of a terminal disease are gardening, spending time in the wilderness, and exploring the inner wilderness of the unconscious with psychedelics—all of which would have served a similar role for our ancestors going back at least to the origins of agriculture in the Neolithic and perhaps to the tending of populations of wild plants by humans and other hominins long before then. (Our earliest evidence of the existence of death rituals comes from a bouquet of Yarrow flowers buried with the body of a Neanderthal child in what is now Iraq. This strikes me—the significance of honoring the dead with the offering of a plant that facilitates the healthy flow of blood in the body when it is alive.)

In an era of electric lights and reliable indoor heat (for those who can afford them) and a global economic system that keeps the same foods reliably on the supermarket shelves of wealthy nations throughout the year, we are no longer immersed in those rhythms unless we make a conscious choice to be.

Our disconnection with the sun in and of itself creates major disruptions in our internal rhythms. We are beings of light and darkness as much as we are beings of earth, air, fire, and water. Gil Hedley points out that the cranium is translucent around the eyes, allowing light to reach the pineal gland, which plays a central role in regulating sleep and dreaming. Our skin is translucent, too, allowing light to penetrate into our fascia. He explained this to an interviewer (Waters 2015):

> *When the Periodic Chart of the Elements was being developed, the discovery of the elements was a process involving light. The elements have characteristic absorption and emission spectra which can be discerned by interpretation with a spectroscope. Whether carbon, hydrogen, nitrogen, oxygen, or the rest, the elements alone and in combination emit light. The human body, comprised of these elements, is a light emitting, light*

absorbing phenomenon, and this is an aspect of our human anatomy that we might do well to consider in our quest for self understanding and health. I am fond of saying that "the human body" is not limited by the boundaries of our skin. We are all part of one human body, and the sun is a shared organ, our "master gland."

Victor Anderson spoke of the sun as the god of our solar system because its light and heat and gravity and electromagnetic winds shape everything that happens here.

The identification of seasonal affective disorder and the success of treatments for it—vitamin D-3, full spectrum light, and that most solar of plants, St. John's Wort, which blooms at midsummer, when the sun is at its peak—have brought some awareness to the role of the sun in mental health. Just as important as sunlight, though, is darkness, and the dreaming we do within that darkness.

Traditionally, in many parts of the world, the dark months of the year were a time of telling certain stories around the fire that could only be told after the first frost or the first snow and the long nights of dreaming. Storytelling and dreaming are both ways that we metabolize experiences and emotions in ways that give us just enough removal from the original situation to be able to process them more fully: stories allow us to see someone else go through experiences we might have shared, letting us recontexualize those experiences without completely reliving them. Dreams allow us to repeat and complete sensations and emotions that remain unresolved from waking life. We are also more receptive to the whispers of the Otherworld when we are dreaming.

Sleep is also the time when our liver does most of its work of metabolizing the hormones that have circulated through our blood throughout the day (as well as anything the body doesn't want to assimilate or re-assimilate). Chinese medicine likens the work of the liver to a cleansing wind. Subhuti Dharmananda writes, "The liver is the source of wind. The wind disperses the water vapors and clouds and lets spaces develop, through which the great *yang,* the sun, can shine and the wood can grow. The penetrating and reflecting light enters through the eyes and the images then restrain or agitate the wind."

Wind is always in motion, and this clearing and cleansing of the liver is also a function of the Cauldron of Motion. The element of wood—the element of new growth in spring—is also housed in and associated with the liver in Daoist medicine. The wood *yang* is the ability to advance toward our goals, the wood *yin* is the ability to relax and withdraw. The quality of the liver's function is felt in the second position on the wrist (two fingers down from the scaphoid) in Chinese pulse diagnosis, and this is one of the ways I assess what is happening within the Cauldron of Motion. The deepest level of the pulse there tells me what impact processing past events has had on the liver, the middle depth tells me how the liver is processing the past right now, and the level closest to the surface tells me how the liver feels about what it is about to begin responding to.

Sleep and water are what the liver needs most—water to allow for flow, sleep to allow for time when the internal wind is not being influenced by new information pouring in through the eyes. Alcohol and most pharmaceuticals force the liver to work hard to process the poison they represent (and sometimes purposeful poisoning is necessary to stop even more harmful processes, so pharmaceuticals are not universally unhealthy choices) and will disrupt the liver's processing—and since the liver's physical processing of hormones is integral to our emotional processing through dreaming, they disrupt our emotional processing too.

Reishi is one of my favorite allies for helping people process things through dreaming. I learned about this years ago when someone came to me for panic attacks that had begun suddenly, in the wake of big life changes. I gave her a formula that included Reishi to settle the heart. She came back a few weeks later and said that the panic attacks were less frequent and that in her dreams, she had been meeting with people she had unfinished business with and bringing old situations to resolution, so I continued her on that formula. A few weeks later she came back and said that everything was great, but that she was waking up feeling like she had done too much work in her dreams. So we took the Reishi out, and the dream meetings stopped. Later, she wanted to resume that dream work, so I added Reishi back in, and sure enough, the dreams returned.

For people who wake from dreams startled and agitated, I like to combine Reishi with Schizandra and Motherwort. When that waking is sudden and fearful, I give a single drop of Wormwood.

What we don't metabolize, we hold on to. Since communication within our bodies is facilitated by water and lipids conducting chemical and electrical signals, this tends to present in the form of stagnant, swampy conditions, with tissues bogged down with metabolic waste that blocks circulation.

Stifled emotions that are still fresh or are swiftly remobilized tend to present as anger, manic laughter, or the hot tears of sudden sorrow. Think of the heat you can feel beneath the surface of a compost pile, the heat of a continuous process that is blocked from finding its way out into the world. I treat these kind of resurfacing hot emotions the same way I treat hyperreactivity: with bitter, cooling mints like Lemon Balm, Motherwort, and Skullcap; the cooling flowers of Rose and Hawthorn; and plants that release tension to allow the heat to flow through (something we will soon discuss at great length.)

But some emotions, particularly grief, tend to settle into the watery places in the body, especially the lungs and the fascia. They bog us down and often have the dull, aching quality of rheumatic pains—your soul can feel the way an arthritic person's bones and joints feel just before a rainstorm. The body needs help clearing them. Bitter, warming, aromatic herbs can accomplish this well—their bitterness stimulates the liver, the heat stimulates the circulation, and the aromatic quality opens and engages the mind and the senses.

In the early stages of such malaise, kitchen herbs like Basil, Rosemary, Onion, and Sage can be helpful, as can teas and steams of evergreen needles. When I lived on the West Coast, I would always have fresh Red Cedar boughs present in the room when working with a grieving person and would encourage grieving people to burn dried Cedar leaves at home. Now that

I am back in Maine, I use the needles, resin, and cones of White Pine for steams to open the lungs and move recent, fresh grief. Burning Frankincense can help raise the spirits in such times as well.

When grief has lingered longer, stronger medicines are needed. Most are roots that grow in damp places: Angelica, Elecampane, Eastern and Western Skunk Cabbage. They clear the grief held in the lungs and open the airways to allow the breath of life to enter again. Black Cohosh helps to ease this kind of stagnant depression by allowing the cerebrospinal fluid to detoxify the brain—when we stew in the same old neurotransmitters we stew in the same old emotions. Calamus relights the fire of expression, allowing us to burn through the fog and give voice to the deepest truths that rise up through us.

The folk medicine of disparate cultures throughout the world's northern latitudes long recognized the need to move the inner waters during the transitions between the dark and bright times of the year. The Birch sap that rises as spring approaches and spring greens like Dandelions, Cleavers, Violets, and Nettles were welcomed as foods that would "purify the blood" by helping the liver, the kidneys, and the lymph carry metabolic waste out of the body after long months of being confined indoors and eating heavy foods.

When autumn came, people would go through another round of purification, so they would not be carrying so much heaviness that it would wear them down as they entered the dark of the year. From the Bronze Age into the late nineteenth century, people in Ireland, like their counterparts in North America, Scandinavia, and Siberia, would seek the aid of fire and darkness in preparing them for winter. In Ireland, people built peat fires in stone chambers and sealed up the entrance, staying inside for hours, coming out occasionally to plunge in water. The name for this kind of chamber was *teach alais*—the sweat house.

We have only nineteenth-century accounts to go on to understand the nature of this ritual. Those texts, written by English-speaking people describing what they heard and observed among people in the countryside, tell us that the sweat houses were mainly used to treat rheumatism and that women would occasionally put Kelp on the fire to aid their complexions.

Is it possible that the ritual had a deeper significance as well? I would say that it is almost certain that it did, though we will likely never know, because people in an occupied country whose native language had been outlawed were unlikely to tell even sympathetic interviewers from the occupying culture about remnant ancestral spiritual practices. But everywhere else where such rituals are performed, they serve—or originally served—the purpose of spiritual purification. And where ritual forms are the same, ritual functions tend to be as well. (At the very least, in the early forms of the ritual.) Darkness has a way of turning the mind inward, and aromatic smoke like that of a peat fire puts people into a receptive state, heat stirs the blood, and sweat helps release the memories the body holds. The Irish frame drum, the *bodhrán*, and the haunting sounds of *sean -nós* singing, the trance-based vocal style of Ireland's Gaeilge-speaking West, may have played a role in further facilitating shifts in consciousness that would allow access to the guidance of the Otherworld. It is also significant that this would have been a ritual of going naked into the darkness during the time of year when the ancestors and the Daoine Sidhe are said to walk most closely with us.

We know that the Irish had extensive contact with Scandinavian people, sometimes as adversaries and sometimes as trading partners, and they likely also had contact with the Indigenous peoples of the areas that are now New England and Canada's Maritime Provinces. The Tuath Dé, the Tribe of the Gods, are said to have been people who left Ireland to go to the North and returned bearing magic and knowledge, which they took with them beneath the hollow hills, the ancient burial mounds, when they left this world. Later sages, poets, and saints were said to have sailed to lands far to the West and returned bearing the fruits of the visions they experienced there. Cross-pollination of ritual and medicinal techniques among all the people of northern latitudes seems more a certainty than a possibility.

All of this brings us to the nature of the third and final cauldron—the Cauldron of Wisdom.

The Cauldron of Wisdom is inverted in us when we are born, and it remains inverted throughout most people's lives. Its waters are the waters of the infinite—just as in the Cauldron of Incubation, just as in the Otherworld Well. For most people, those waters flow down through the Cauldron of Motion, with more and more wisdom being retained as engaging joy and sorrow turns that middle cauldron more and more upright. Many people, however, never do the necessary work for the Cauldron of Motion to be turned from its initial position—tilted on its side—with the result that the water from the Cauldron of Wisdom spills out and is lost. I experience this cauldron as the electric blue of the sky just before dawn and of the center of the flame. It doesn't show up in the pulse directly, but I can often feel elements of its influence on the Cauldron of Motion in the layer of the pulse closest to the surface and in the first pulse position on the left wrist, the position just below the scaphoid, which is connected with the heart in Chinese pulse diagnosis.

Then there are the *filidh*, the poets (singular: *fili*), who turn the Cauldron of Wisdom upward and light a fire beneath it. Poetry was not just a form of personal expression in ancient Ireland, especially for the *filidh*. Erynn Rowan Laurie tells: "The word *fili* probably means 'seer.' The word derives from the Archaic Irish **weis* by way of the Insular Celtic word **wel-* which had the original imperative meaning "see!" or "look at!" and is related to the Irish verb *to be*. Their work included divination, blessing and blasting magic, creating praise poetry for their patrons, the preservation of lore and genealogies, and occasionally the rendering of judgments. *Cormac's Glossary* derives *fili* from "*fi*, 'poison' in satire, and *li*, 'splendor' in praise, and it is variously that the poet proclaims."

Poetry is the language of the Human Self that comes closest to expressing the Animal Self's experience of its encounters with the living world, the Otherworld, and the divine. Its imagery invokes the presence of plants, animals, ancestors, and forces of nature. Its rhythm induces trance. Its sounds evoke emotion. A properly trained *fili* had the power to speak words that could heal or could harm and the power to write withering words that would take away the power of a corrupt or brutal chieftain or king. The greatest poetry speaks to all three selves and calls them into alignment. It comes from the root, out of the Cauldron of Incubation, moves upward through the Cauldron of Motion, and then, if the Cauldron of Motion is fully upright and all the conditions are right, it blazes up as a fire in the head that warms the now upright Cauldron of Wisdom and pours forth as "a terrifying stream of speech from the mouth."

Such poetry emerges during a state of *imbas*, "poetic frenzy," cultivated through time in the wilderness, *scrying* (divinatory gazing) in lakes and wells, immersion in darkness, and other techniques of shifting consciousness. This may have included the ingestion of visionary medicines like the ones we will discuss in chapter 5. A fascinating, if highly speculative, book by the late Peter Lamborn Wilson called *Ploughing the Clouds* makes an intriguing case that the ancient Irish, like some other northern peoples, may have used the iconic red and white *Amanita muscaria* mushroom for ritual purposes (1999). Erynn Rowan Laurie and Timothy White make a similar argument, more cautiously and more convincingly, in their essay "Speckled Snake, Brother of Birch" (n.d.). Among other things, they suggest that descriptions of *filidh* eating raw flesh from the mounds of the Sidhe may have been an oblique reference to harvesting and eating the mushroom—which, like Reishi, is the red, vital, fruiting body of a fungus that emerges from the white mycelium of an organism that feeds off dying roots and rotting leaves and other decaying matter. So to eat of the flesh of such a mushroom truly would be to partake of something of the Otherworld. (It also can be a good way to unintentionally become a permanent denizen of the Otherworld—*Amanita muscaria* is toxic at the wrong dosage or in the wrong preparation, and bears a close resemblance to even more toxic mushrooms which can kill through rapid induction of liver failure. Modern psychonauts who are not also mycologists would do well to stick with the gentler mushrooms of the *Psilocybe* genus that sprout up in pastures as Samhain approaches.)

Describing the state the *filidh* would enter, Laurie writes: "The translation of the word *imbas* as 'poetic frenzy' is not an overstatement of the condition. This Celtic form of enlightenment is no gentle melding with the oneness of the universe. Instead, it is a passionate, sometimes uncontrollable engagement with the fabric of reality. The energies accessed when all the cauldrons are turned into their upright positions does indeed feel like fire flowing through the head, expanding, quickening, and burning, as when Amirgen proclaimed 'I am a God who shapes fire for a head.' "

This is the true definition of an ecstatic state. Though, as Amirgen himself tells us, great and pure joy can lead to ecstasy, ecstasy is not joy, and while it has elements of bliss it also has elements of terror. "Ecstasy" is derived from the Greek word *ekstasis,* "displacement, distraction, astonishment, entrancement." Navigating this state takes great skill and great focus.

Celtic traditions, both Gaelic traditions like those of Ireland and Scotland and Brythonic traditions like those of Cornwall, Wales, and Brittany, are full of warnings that encounters with the Otherworld, especially encounters that occur at powerful places or powerful times of year, will render a person "mad, dead, or a poet." The training of the *filidh* prepared them to resolve madness into poetry before it could kill them. But to encounter the Otherworld was also to touch death and to be forever transformed in ways that may make you seem mad to the rest of the culture and will definitely make the rest of the culture seem mad to you.

The nature of such an encounter with the Otherworld is described by an Irish legend, the Vision of Óengus. Óengus Óg was the son of the Dagda, the "Good God," whose cauldron of plenty fed all of his people, and he was trained by Manannán Mac Lir, the powerful and mysterious god of wild waters who had already been in Ireland when the Tuath Dé arrived and who instructed them in magic, poetry, and music (which, from an ancient perspective, are really all one and the same.) The Dagda made his home in an ancient burial mound at the mouth of the Boyne. This mound would—through the clever wordplay Óengus learned from Manannán—become Óengus's home.

Later, this mound became the place where Manannán gathered the people when it was time for them to leave this world for the Otherworld. He divided the ancient burial mounds spread across Ireland, which are the entrance to that realm, among the departing people as they became the Daoine Sidhe, the fairie people, the People of the Mound. The Boyne is the river that mirrors the Milky Way, and both have their source in the Otherworld Well.

It was in that mound, by that river—in the time when the Tuath Dé still lived and breathed as we do—that Óengus had a dream in which a woman of unearthly beauty appeared beside his bedside. When he went to reach for her hand she vanished. When Óengus woke, an illness was upon him. He did not eat that day. That night he went to bed and dreamed the same dream. Nothing in his waking life could compare to the splendor of this vision. And so it was for two years. (It is also worth noting that all of these symptoms would be consistent with regular ingestion of *Amanita muscaria*, which might have been possible to do without getting even sicker in a time when people's livers were less challenged by environmental toxins, though it would never be wise from a mental health standpoint.)

Across cultures we see the same basic story repeated: a person's true vision awakens in dream, and they cannot rest until they have understood how to integrate what they witnessed in that dream, and they become sick, often to the point of death. In the process, they either waste away and die, go mad, or learn to view and experience the world in a new way, a way that perceives and weaves with the threads of time and space themselves. Mad, dead, or a poet, indeed.

Desperate to heal his son's illness, the Dagda sent people to search the land for the woman from his son's dream. He learned that her name was Caer Ibormeith and she lived in Connacht, a rocky province ruled by Queen Meadbh, who, like Manannán, had been in Ireland before the coming of the Tuath Dé—and who often returned after their departure. Queen Meadbh was known for coming to test the worthiness of those who would be chieftains and kings by appearing to them as an old hag and asking them to make love to her—if they assented, she transformed into a young woman, and in the union with her, the man who would be king was wedded to the land. As we shall see shortly, like her queen, Caer treasured her sovereignty and tested her suitor's willingness to honor it.

Caer Ibormeith's name has great significance. *Caer* means "berry" in Irish Gaeilge (oddly, the same word means "fortress" in Welsh), and *ibormeith* refers to the Yew tree. The berries and leaves of the Yew are highly toxic, causing cardiac and respiratory failure—stilling the Cauldron of Motion. (Yes, as some of you may be aware, a substance from the Pacific Yew is used in treating some forms of breast cancer—but, remember, chemotherapy is an art of administering poison in precisely the right manner and dosage to kill cancer cells without killing the entire organism.) The tree itself is so ancient as to seem immortal. When it grows old, its branches become hollow, suggesting a passage to the Otherworld. When the tree becomes too heavy with age, it can split its trunk without risking disease or facture. It also has an interesting reproductive strategy: it chooses from year to year whether to grow reproductive structures we humans designate as masculine or feminine according to what its community needs, hence it is a shape-shifter. Because of these qualities, Yew is associated with ancestral magic and the magic of the dead—in other words, the powers of the Otherworld. It is for this reason that Yew trees are found in many church cemeteries across areas of Europe where Celtic tribes once lived—those cemeteries were dug on ground already consecrated as burial grounds by the Indigenous cultures that lived there and blessed with the presence of the Yew.

Caer had strong magic of her own. When the Dagda tried to force her father to give her hand in marriage to Óengus, her father replied that he could not compel her to marry anyone for her power was greater than his own. She had the power to transform from the form of a woman to that of a Swan or from the form of a Swan into that of a woman at Samhain. To court her, Óengus would have to meet her at the water's edge when Samhain came around again.

The Old Irish text, as translated by Jeffrey Gantz in his book *Early Irish Myths and Sagas* (1988), tells us what happened the following Samhain:

> *[Óengus] went to Loch Bél Dracon, and there he saw the three fifties of white birds, with silver chains, and golden hair about their heads.*

74

Oengus was in human form at the edge of the lake, and he called to the
girl, saying "Come and speak with me, Cáer!" "Who is calling to me?"
asked Cáer. "Oengus is calling," he replied. "I will come," she said, "if you
promise me that I may return to the water." "I promise that," he said.
She went to him, then: he put his arms round her, and they slept in the
form of swans until they had circled the lake three times. Thus, he kept his
promise. They left in the form of two white birds and flew to Bruig ind
Maicc Oic [Óengus's habitation at the mouth of the Boyne], and there
they sang until the people inside fell asleep for three days and three nights.

This part of the story is remarkable on several levels: in order to meet
Caer in the fullness of her power, Óengus had to himself become a Swan.
When they first made love, and when they traveled home, they did so in bird
form. When they arrived, together they sang the incantations that put all
present into the kind of deep sleep that was ritually used for the incubation
of visions.

One thing that connects the *filidh* with the shamans of other cultures is
that they wore cloaks made of feathers—and in the case of the *filidh*, those
were cloaks of Swan feathers. A Swan travels three realms—the earth, the
heavens, and the waters. Óengus's wedding was also an initiation.

I have been beautifully haunted by this story since childhood, when, as a
precocious eight-year-old, I first read William Butler Yeats's liberally interpreted poetic retelling of the beginning of the story—"The Song of Wandering Aengus" (1897, 1899, 1991).

Yeats's original working title for his was poem "A Mad Song," which
points to the thin, thin line between the visionary fervor of ecstatic frenzy
and true psychosis. The poem begins with the words:

I went out to a hazel wood
Because a fire was in my head.

Every time I read those lines, I feel a spark of that fire leap into me.
The fire in the head compels us to go into the forest to reconnect with the

wholeness of who we are. To do that, we must first slip the constraints of this culture, and the madness those constraints can bring once the fire has begun to burn.

What wild spring rises through me?
What strange fire burns in my heart?

Though snow flutters like white moths on the wing
and the rolling hills are sleeping Swans beneath a starry sky
the buds of the Cottonwood swell,
the sap rises in the Maple and the Birch,

and deep within a tight, tight bud
the Apple blossom waits
to send its scent
to guide me home in springtime

before the mountainside blooms.

4

OF PAN AND PANIC

The ancient Greeks spoke of a wild man with the legs and horns of a goat who dwelt in the forests and hills beyond the city walls and the village edge. Sometimes when the wind was right, you could catch his strange music and his musky scent drifting through the air, calling you to a wild dance.

They said that to encounter Pan was to risk madness, that his music induced *panikon*, which simply means "panic," in the hearts of villagers and the city folk.

Hidden beneath that warning is a deeper truth: you only experience panic if you resist the wild dance. You force your muscles to tense—but your Animal Self wants to move with the music. Your thwarted desire does not die down; it pushes against the tension, forcing the movement—and the amplification—of the fear you locked into your muscles when you decided to resist the call to dance.

In the Irish tradition we see those experiencing great violence and trauma fleeing to the wilderness for refuge. Most striking perhaps is the story of one of the last Pagan kings in Ireland, Suibhne Geilt, known in English as Mad Sweeney. (*Geilt,* Irish Gaeilge for "madness," is derived from a proto-Celtic word for "wildness." It is also the term for a class of ecstatic poets who spent time alone in the wilderness in order to be able to allow the fire in their heads to blaze freely.) To put the story in its simplest terms, Suibhne was cursed by a saint for fighting back against the construction of a Christian church on his family's sacred land, when next he went into battle he was driven mad by the sounds of war and fled into the wilderness. In that time, Ireland was covered with great forests of Oak and Hazel, and Suibhne grew feathers and leapt from tree to tree.

When the madness passed through him, he came back from the forest and became a monk. Some of the greatest lyric poetry in the Irish language is written from the point of view of the elderly Brother Suibhne remembering his time in the forest. The late Irish poet and Nobel Laureate Seamus Heaney does better than anyone else writing in English to capture the spirit of the original Gaeilge text (2001). In one particularly striking passage, Sweeney, as Heaney calls him, describes how he forsook the call of the trumpet, sound of the hunt and of battle, for the trumpeting of the Stag, the great Red Deer, symbol of sovereignty and kingship in Pagan Ireland:

I prefer the re-
echoing of the belling of a Stag
among the peaks
to that arrogant horn,

Those unharnessed runners
from glen to glen!
Nobody tames
that royal blood,
each one aloof
on its rightful summit,
antlered, watchful.

The Irish word for "Stag" is *fia fierann,* which is related to the words *fiáin,* which means "wild," and *fear,* "man." The Red Deer is actually an Elk and the Red Deer Stag has the same bugling voice as the male North American Elk. The English call the Red Deer Stag the Roebuck. Pagan kingship in Ireland was rooted in being wedded to the land and carried the obligation to defend the vulnerable in the same way that the Stag protects the herd. I gained a visceral understanding of this when first I met the Red Deer.

In the forests and fields above Lough Leane in Killarney (Cuille Airne, "Church of the Blackthorn Berry"), in the shadow of the castle where the *taoisigh* (chieftains) of my clan lived, some of the last descendants of the original native herds of Red Deer lived.

In autumn, the Red Deer Stags gather branches and lichen and moss to crown their antlers—in the time of rutting, and in the time of the Deer hunt, they engage in ritual combat. The Stag who emerges victorious becomes the locus of power within the herd, its protector.

In the weeks before the rutting season began, I traveled to the remnant forest those herds call home, seeking to understand the ways of my ancestors. I prayed beneath an Oak at the edge of a field, and then rounded the bend to a thicket, where a Stag came out to meet me—barrel-chested and with antlers as wide as my arm span. He raised his head high and cantered across the field—first showing his power, then trying to lead me away from the herd, and then circling it to mark a protective boundary.

I sat still, and soon he did too, resting beneath a tree while the does and the younger bucks grazed. In the way of the wild, when he knew his kin were safe, he relaxed into calm presence.

I understood then that it was the Stag who taught us what a chieftain was—not the other way around. This was the authentic expression of sovereignty that Suibhne tried to hold on to in the face of the model of leadership that came in with Christianity—a model that sought to make the king and the chieftain enforcers of the rigid laws in a book written in a distant desert, as interpreted by Latin-speaking theologians. The restriction imposed by those laws was an insult to Suibhne's soul, and his soul rebelled against that restriction, driving him into the wilderness.

There is an interesting parallel in the story of Mis, daughter of a king named Dair (*dair* is an Irish word for "Oak"), who was driven mad with grief when she found her father's severed head on the battlefield. She fled into the mountains that now bear her name and grew claws and long hair and defended her freedom ferociously. She was brought back to the world of humans by the patience, tenderness, and music of a harpist who went into the mountains to court her. (Sharon Blackie retells the story beautifully in *If Women Rose Rooted* [2019].)

I have always found that when the life of this culture becomes too brutal and restricting for me, time in the forest allows my terror or rage or grief to have room to flow freely until, emptied of my pain, I can allow the scent of Spruce and Pine, the drumming of the Pileated Woodpecker, and the call of the Loons from the lake below to call me back to myself. I have known many veterans who have found healing from the ravages of war by spending time in the wilderness, outside the restrictions and expectations of the society that sent them to see and do and experience things that those at home do not want to know about.

In a lecture, John Moriarty said that a psychosis is bigger than the universe that contains it. One way of dealing with that reality is to carefully and deliberately loosen the boundaries that the Human Self's beliefs place on the Animal Self's experiences, and then let the Animal Self have the space to run free. From Suibhne Geilt to John the Baptist, the wilderness has long been the refuge of those whose vision and passion could not be contained by the structures and strictures of society. Attempting to resist the call of such visions and stirrings courts even greater madness than following them.

Wilhelm Reich understood anxiety and trauma in similar terms—and saw them as endemic to modern life. Reich's teacher and mentor Sigmund Freud saw the human body as animated by the libido, the personal erotic drive. Eros in the original Greek sense referred to the drive to live. Freud saw the libido primarily in sexual terms, narrowly and literally defined. He believed that civilization depended on the taming and subjugation of this force and that a healthy culture was the result of the redirection of the libido.

Reich saw the libido manifested in a physical force, which he called *orgone*, which flowed through the body from the core to the periphery. He believed this energy was one and the same as sexual energy, but that its function was not limited to the realms we would define as "sexual." He saw this force, in fact, as the driving force of life itself, the "vegetative energy" that was expressed not only in the full and free expression of a liberated human being but also in the sprouting of a seed, the Dolphin's joyous leaping from the sea, the electricity of a lightning storm, the dance of the aurora borealis, the blazing of the sun, and the swirling life of the galaxy. He wrote, "since the life process and the sexual process are one and the same, it goes without saying that the sexual, vegetative energy is active in everything that lives" (1973).

Reich shared his teacher's belief that this civilization as we know it depends on the subjugation of that erotic force, but he believed that repression was harmful. He saw that repression as something that created physiological tension that blocked the flow of *orgone* through the body and saw that obstruction as the root of most modern mental and physical illness. He understood anxiety as the consequence of upwelling energy in the body being blocked by tension and reanimating the fear that had created the tension in the first place.

From a biological standpoint, our muscles constrict when we receive a signal from our limbic system—that ancient part of the brain that warns us when we face an impending threat. Our muscles tense to prepare to deliver or receive a blow—or to run away.

When the threatening situations we experience remain unresolved, as most of the stressful situations in contemporary life do, we remain constricted.

Tension serves not only to help us brace against experiences but also to neutralize, numb, or sequester sensory and emotional memories. Herbalist jim mcdonald notes that "tension or spasm in tissues impedes the flow of the circulation and the body's vital force." Where blood flows, awareness goes.

Where the flow of blood is cut off, so is awareness. Cutting off awareness by restricting blood flow is one of the body's brilliant strategies for helping us continue to act when we are in seemingly impossible situations. It prevents us from being completely awash in unbearable sensations and memories.

Reich observed the effects of chronic tension, and its impediment to the flow of the vital force in his patients. "If the layer of rigidified conflicts were especially numerous and functioned automatically, if they formed a compact, not easily penetrable unity, the patient felt them as an 'armor' surrounding the living organism. The armor could lie on the 'surface' or in the 'depth,' could be 'as soft as a sponge' or 'as hard as a rock.' Its function in every case was to protect the person against unpleasurable experiences. However, it also entailed a reduction in the organism's capacity for pleasure" (1978).

Reich, who watched and spoke out against the rise of fascism in Europe before fleeing to the United States, saw that this armoring both reinforced and was reinforced by cultures of cruelty, violence, and rigid control. "The character structure of modern man, who reproduces a six-thousand-year-old patriarchal authoritarian culture is typified by characterological armoring against his inner nature and against the social misery which surrounds him. This characterological armoring of the character is the basis of isolation, indigence, craving for authority, fear of responsibility, mystic longing, sexual misery, and neurotically impotent rebelliousness."

If you cannot feel the pulsing of life at your own core, how can you feel the flow of life in a forest stream and understand that it is related to the flow of life within you? If you cannot feel your own sorrow or pain, how can you feel another's? Cutting off sensation cuts off empathy. Early in the Cold War, Robert Jay Lifton, a psychiatrist who worked with soldiers who had committed atrocities, coined the phrase "psychic numbing" to refer to the way in which the psyche fragments in order to keep the core persona from experiencing the horrors it is participating in. He later documented the ways in which psychic numbing can take place across entire societies, describing the ways in which people in the United States continued life as usual in the face of the threat of nuclear annihilation (Lifton and Falk 1991). Buddhist psychologist, activist, and writer Joanna Macy has developed a repertoire of practices called "The Work That Reconnects" that seeks to reawaken and reintegrate the numbed parts of our psyches through meditation and rituals that reconnect us with the beauty and fragility of human and other-than-human life (Macy and Brown 2014).

No amount of psychic numbing can shut us down permanently and completely. When life, as it will, stirs within that armor and pushes against it, the armored person, who viscerally believes that their armor is the one thing protecting them from the world (and the world from their own instincts and desires) experiences profound anxiety. Reich saw that the solution to this was releasing that armoring, which would restore healthy flow to the system.

In many ways, Reich's approach aligns with ideas of traditional Western herbalism. Going back to the time of the ancient Greeks, Western herbal traditions have spoken of a vital force that animates the body and moves from the core to the periphery. These traditions have seen the herbalist's role as using plants to support the flow of that vital force. A classic example lies in the tendency of clinical herbalists and folk herbalists alike to see a fever as a healthy rallying of the vital force to drive out infection—a position that is increasingly shared by modern biomedicine. Rather than suppressing the fever with cooling herbs, herbalists tend to use herbs that release tension to relax the muscles and allow the blood to flow out to the periphery, so that it opens the pores, allowing the body to sweat and release excess heat.

What is anxiety but a psychic fever trying to move through a body that will not give it full expression? Yet most herbalists today try to subdue anxiety using large doses of herbs that dampen brain activity by the same mechanism—stimulation of the GABA receptors—as pharmaceutical anxiety medications. In my practice, I have found much better results by giving people herbs that release tension and encouraging them to let the anxiety move. Usually I begin cautiously, with a slow release of tension, to keep people from getting overwhelmed. Sometimes it is necessary to use some subtly cooling herbs to calm an over-reactive nervous system, but here I prefer to use Rose family plants like Hawthorn (*Crataegus* spp.) that reduce hyper-reactivity or small doses of bitter mints like Skullcap (*Scutellaria* spp.) that bring awareness down into the body by stimulating the enteric nervous system rather than large doses of GABAergic herbs like Valerian (*Valeriana* spp.). (The bitter mints do tend to have GABAergic activity in higher doses, so I like to keep the dose low unless I am dealing with quieting the effects of physiological nerve pain.) The GABA system is complex, and there are good reasons for engaging it directly, but doing it in a blunt force way is like icing an injury—it may bring some potential relief, but it will slow healing.

I learned the importance of that slow release several summers ago, when I was beginning to get to know a few of the many species of the *Pedicularis* genus, plants with an amazing gift for relaxing muscular tension. When I am getting to know a plant, I often act like an awkward and overly enthusiastic teenager with a crush and end up trying to immerse myself in everything related to that plant.

So it was, that August, when I became infatuated with *Pedicularis*. I went into the mountains with a friend and found a beautiful streambed lined with *Pedicularis racemosa*—delicate plants with ethereal white flowers. For every three of the plants that I put into a mason jar for tincturing, I ate one or two. By late afternoon, my world was shimmering. Leaving the streambed, we found a stand of *Pedicularis groenlandica* dried out in the sun, and I decided to take some of that species home as well.

The next morning, I filled the bathtub with *Pedicularis groenlandica*, and, while I soaked, I took a big dose of a *Pedicularis bracteosa* tincture someone had sent me. When I got out of the bath, I went to an acupuncture session. I told the acupuncturist that I wanted to release tension. So she needled Kidney 1, a point known as the "bubbling spring."

Now, most people find the stimulation of Kidney 1 to be deeply ground-ing. What I did not know at the time, and what that acupuncturist may or may not have known, is that the spring can bubble in different directions. Usually people feel the spring—the energy being moved—draining down-ward, carrying tension out through the bottom of their feet. But the spring can also bubble upward, stirring up the emotion that the tension has held in.

That is what happened to me that day. After the appointment, I sobbed for six hours straight.

I was lucky in some ways, because I understood most of what happened—I knew that as tension was releasing, emotion built up behind it. I was fine. Mostly. For better or worse, I tend to be someone who goes for big, cathartic releases. But I knew that not everyone would emerge from that kind of experience okay. Especially if they did not have a framework for understanding what they were experiencing.

What kinds of plants release tension? Plants that engage the parasympathetic. When we speak of anxiety, fear, anger, terror, and wild grief, we tend to speak of the activation of the sympathetic response—the fight-or-flight response. But what is actually happening is the disengagement of the parasympathetic response. In the absence of the connective instincts represented by the parasympathetic, the sympathetic tries to drive and focus us toward dealing with an external threat in an urgent and single-minded way. If we have faced similar threats before, we default to whatever response kept us from being killed in the past.

When we re-engage the parasympathetic, we reorient ourselves in time and place. If we discover that we are actually safe, we become calm, and the nervous system begins finding another way to respond to the stimulus that triggered our fear. If this happens early enough in the process and is repeated frequently enough in similar situations, eventually our brains will eventually reinterpret the meaning of the associated sensations in more benign terms.

If we discover we are not actually safe in that moment but are able to regain a grounded, embodied presence through re-engaging the parasympathetic, we will instinctively seek out more connective ways to resolve the situation—through negotiation or through seeking help from others.

There are three kinds of plants that I seek out in these situations. Each engages the parasympathetic slightly differently—acrid-tasting plants, bitter plants, and aromatic plants.

The swiftest and strongest parasympathetic reset comes from acrid-tasting plants. The acrid taste is a burning sensation experienced in the back of the throat at a point where the vagus nerve meets the tissues of the esophagus. Many plant and fungal alkaloids taste acrid. Some steroidal or triterpenoid saponins, including some cardiac glycosides are acrid as well. Lobeline from *Lobelia* species can be considered the archetypal acrid compound. The strong signal sent along the ventral branch of the vagus nerve awakens and connects all of our primary nerve centers—those in the pelvis, solar plexus, heart, and brain—instantly reorienting us. This reactivates the parasympathetic response and results in an immediate relaxation of tension, opening and deepening of the breath and dilation of the blood vessels, bringing oxygenated blood, and hence awareness, back to areas cut off from circulation and sensation by constriction. This allows new signals to travel to and from all of our organs (except the adrenal medulla, the sole internal organ not innervated by nerves branching from the vagus and the organ whose influence becomes strongest when the vagal signal is at its weakest). Stimulate the acrid taste receptor too strongly, and you can make someone throw up. But sometimes that vomiting can be cathartic, helping a person have a visceral experience of releasing something poisonous that had entered into their body.

Strongly bitter plants can have a similar effect through a different mechanism. All terpenes and all alkaloids have some degree of bitterness. The bitter taste is first experienced on the tongue, where a pair of cranial nerves carry it to the amygdala, which signals the liver and gall bladder to begin secreting bile, the stomach to release its digestive secretions, and the mouth to begin to salivate, all of which can only occur through parasympathetic engagement. This digestive stimulation also brings awareness down out of the head and into the solar plexus. Extremely bitter compounds—mostly alkaloids, but some terpenes as well—also have a strong action on the bitter taste receptors in the respiratory tract and the lower digestive tract (and possibly in the heart, if they pass into the bloodstream in sufficient quantities). Very, very bitter plants like Gentian and Wormwood can bring about a strong reset response throughout the nervous system, much as acrid plants do. The extreme bitterness of the mescaline in San Pedro and Peyote cacti and the plants used to make Ayahuasca may be partially responsible for preparing the body to become more open to sensations as the brain becomes more open to new sensory input, allowing for a more dramatic kind of neurological reset, which we will talk more about soon. That extreme bitterness is definitely responsible for the cathartic vomiting those medicines can induce. In the Native American Church, when someone vomits during a ceremony, instead of saying they got sick, they say that person got well. The Native American Church has a better track record of curing people of the poison of alcohol addiction than almost any other group.

Aromatic plants, those rich in the light terpenes and light phenols that allow plants to communicate with each other through the air, are the gentlest relaxants. The olfactory nerve carries the news of their presence to the amygdala, which immediately recognizes it as the sign of the presence of our wild green kindred and activates the parasympathetic so we can receive the messages the plants are bringing.

Plants that engage the parasympathetic bring us back to ourselves and to each other, allowing healing to begin. From there, we can open more deeply to the wild and to the Otherworld as well, which give us new context for reimagining our lives.

They called Suibhne mad
because he preferred
the bugling of the Red Deer

to the sounds of the horn
and the hunt
and fled the company
of his fellow men

for a forest
then so vast
he could leap
from tree to tree.

One footstep
on his wild road
and you too
will find
madness,
or poetry,
or death.

The art lies
in resolving
madness
into poetry
to forestall death.

Dream enough
of the Roebuck
and the robeless king

and you will find yourself
wandering down
an bóthar fiáin,

not noticing
when the path
gives way to a Deer trail
and then the opening
created by the way
roots follow
underground streams

until you kneel down
among the Alders
at the water's edge,
digging Calamus

the fire of its root
lighting the fire at your root
and the fire in your heart
and the fire in your head

which spill forth
from your lips

as you join
in the song
of the Blackbirds

calling the world
to flower
and fruit
and seed
once more.

5

PERILOUS QUESTIONS

There is a story in the Arthurian legends of Wales and Brittany and the West of England that speaks of a king who was wounded in the groin while returning from a war in a foreign land. The wound would not heal.

In the old ways of both Britain and Ireland, a king was wedded to the land, a union as profound as any human union, and a union that was understood in erotic as well as romantic terms. This wounded king could no longer bring life to the land, and so his land became a wasteland. Some versions of the story say that at this time he also failed to defend the women who protected the holy wells from which life and healing flowed and that when those women were killed, the wells stopped giving water.

The only relief the king could find from the pain of his wound came when he sat by the edge of the water, fishing, so he became known as the Fisher King. Despite his suffering, the suffering of his people, and the barrenness of the land, every night the Fisher King held a great banquet in his castle, and every night a grail would appear.

Christian versions of the legend describe this grail as the chalice that holds the blood of Christ, but in older versions of the story, the grail is understood to be the cauldron of Cerridwen, cauldron of life, death, rebirth, and transformation. The grail would have healed the Fisher King if only he or someone in his court would ask the perilous question: "Whom does the grail serve?"

Why was this question perilous? One reason was because of the implications of its answer: the grail served Cerridwen, and in serving her, it served life. The only way for it to bring healing would be for the king to renew his commitment to serving life—renew and make good on his wedding vows to the spirit of the land.

Collectively, like the Fisher King, we too are bleeding at the root, leaking from the Cauldron of Incubation, and unwilling to ask about the nature of what could cure us, because to understand the nature of the medicine would be to understand the nature of the wound, and we would rather numb and cauterize it. Our idea of the individual self, cut off from the web of life from which it arises, insulated from the experience of others, has to die in order for us to be reborn into the knowledge of our connection with all of life, a knowledge that will bring profound responsibility. As a result, we are also cut off from the fullness of life.

In an essay introducing a later edition of *Lady Chatterley's Lover,* the novelist D. H. Lawrence wrote, "We are bleeding at the roots, because we are cut off from the earth and sun and stars, and love is a grinning mockery, because, poor blossom, we plucked it from its stem on the tree of Life, and expected it to keep on blooming in our civilised vase on the table" (2006). If we acknowledge the wound, we would be overcome with the desire to reroot, and that is anathema to our current civilization.

The other reason that the question was a perilous one for the Fisher King was that the grail's source was in the Otherworld, and dealing with the Otherworld is a perilous undertaking for people unfamiliar with its ways or impure in their intentions. Even beneficial knowledge from the Otherworld has the effect of permanently changing our sense of ourselves and our place in this world. And the Otherworld demands respect—a kind of respect few of us grow up learning in a culture that denies that world's very existence. To learn it, we need to look to older ways.

Otherworld knowledge is spoken of in Irish tradition as the province of the Otherworld's denizens: "the Good People," "the Gentry," "the Other Crowd." All names for the Daoine Sidhe, the People of the Mound, the mysterious people who inhabited Ireland in the time before the coming of the Celts. The mythic histories tell us that their arrival and their decline was heralded by the blooming of the Hawthorn trees that grew upon the hollow hills beneath which they disappeared as Celtic culture took hold.

On the morning of Bealtaine, the old celebration of the earth's ecstasy, when the Hawthorn was in bloom, dew shimmering on its blossoms with the splendor of the fine raiments of the Gentry, people would tie ribbons to the tree with prayers for abundance, and hang cloths from its branches that would be saved for use as bandages. But the thorns of the Hawthorn suggested the wrath that would be visited upon any who dared to damage it.

As late as the 1990s, folklorist Eddie Lenihan found many people in the west of Ireland who shared stories of the woes that befell those who damaged Hawthorns: one spoke of the tree beginning to bleed when cut with a crosscut saw, another spoke of a man who, after cutting a Hawthorn, felt thorns in his bed every night for the rest of his life. Those were among the milder consequences associated with such desecration (Lenihan and Green 2004). Such understandings arise from experiencing the world as alive and animated by quite different consciousnesses than our own.

Drawing from her own experiences, Cora Anderson, granddaughter of an herbalist who emigrated from Ireland to Alabama during the Great Hunger, wrote, "The [fairie realm] is not some place put here for the sole benefit of humans. It is teeming with many forms of life, including those who are malevolent and dangerous to humans, not because they are evil but because they are different. They are the wildlife of their native habitat. Most of their antagonism is caused by corruption and destructive behavior toward the environment" (2009).

At the same time, this wild and not-human realm is also the source of folk-healers' knowledge. Throughout rural Ireland, in the time of Cora Anderson's grandfather and beyond, when a person or an animal fell ill, people would send for the "faerie doctor"—someone who had been chosen and trained by the Daoine Sidhe in the ways of working with herbs and other allies in healing and magic. While some today claim to teach that art in weekend workshops, traditionally a person did not choose to undertake that training but rather was abducted or confronted by the Gentry and conscripted into service that would last a lifetime. The initiation into the art was harrowing, and the techniques were fluid, intuitive, and relational, rooted in relationships with the plants, the land, and the Other Crowd. Memorized charms and folk remedies recorded in books today reflect the common knowledge most rural people would have. What each faerie doctor knew arose in the context of their own connections and experiences, and these could not be passed to another verbatim.

One of the best accounts of the work of the fairie doctors comes from the brilliant folklorist, poet, and linguist Lady Jane Wilde (less famous—due to her gender and the times—than her also brilliant son Oscar Fingal O'Fla-hertie Wills Wilde) who enjoyed an unusual level of access to rural Irish culture as a result of her ability to speak the Irish language and her fervent support for Irish freedom. She refers to the dread nature of the ways fairie doctors attained their knowledge and their medicine and the ecstatic state they entered while practicing their craft. In 1888 she wrote:

> *The virtue of herbs is great, but they must be gathered at night, and laid in the hand of a dead man to hold. There are herbs that produce love, and herbs that produce sterility; but only the fairie doctor knows the secrets of their power, and he will reveal the knowledge to no man unless to an adept. The wise women learn the mystic powers from the fairies, but how they pay for the knowledge none dare to tell.*
>
> *The fairy doctors are often seized with trembling while uttering a charm, and look round with a scared glance of terror, as if some awful presence were beside them. But the people have the most perfect faith in the herb-men and wise women, and the faith may often work the cure.*

The Hawthorn is a glyph for the power of the realm whose gate it guards, and to claim the knowledge of some bit of that power out of context invited disaster as surely as harming the Hawthorn did. A woman in the west of Ireland explained this to Lady Augusta Gregory, the great folklorist of the early twentieth century (n.d.):

I knew some could cure with herbs; but it's not right for any one that doesn't understand them to be meddling with them. There was a woman I knew one time wanted a certain herb I knew for a cure for her daughter, and the only place that herb was to be had was down in the bottom of a spring well. She was always asking me would I go and get it for her, but I took advice, and I was advised not to do it. So, then she went herself and she got it out, a very green herb it was, not watercress, but it had a bunch of green leaves. And so soon as she brought it into the house, she fell as if dead and there she lay for two hours. And not long after that she died, but she cured the daughter, and it is well I didn't go to gather the herb, or it's on me all the harm would have come.

The strangeness and perilousness of the path of the faerie doctor stands in sharp contrast to much of the writing and teaching about intuitive herbalism and plant spirit medicine that takes place in our culture today—ways of knowing and being that I have partaken of as student, teacher, and practitioner. The general view is that other-than-human realms are largely benign and that anyone can learn simple techniques to be in contact with them and use the fruits of that labor to improve their own lives and the lives of others. This is an understanding that arises from a culture in which even those who proclaim that the world is alive don't always live in the knowledge of the fullness and literality of that truth—a culture in which knowledge and medicine are commodified and in which most people are used to believing that it is our birthright to have and achieve whatever we desire.

Is the world we inhabit actually less strange and frightening than that of my Irish ancestors? I do not think that it is. If anything, our culture's disrespect for other forms of life has likely heightened the level of antipathy between this world and others. Why, then, do we not see more casualties among people who blunder into the green world unbidden? The answer, I think, is two-fold.

First we need to consider that the baseline from which many of us begin is a place of disconnection from the living world more profound than that of even the most gentrified resident of, say, nineteenth-century Dublin. Think of the questions asked in most quizzes about nature awareness: "Where does your water come from?" "What phase is the moon in right now?" "Name seven wild plants growing where you live." This level of awareness is not only a birthright but also a responsibility for inhabitants of this planet—as is some level of direct experience of the existence of other-than-human minds. The threat the baseline of ignorance within our culture presents to other forms of life makes it in the best interest of the plants and those who honor and protect them to ensure that everyone be brought into the same level of attunement to the world that the average twelve-year-old would have experienced in most places in most parts of history.

The plants do not take kindly toward people trying to storm the gates of knowledge. Daniel Schulke writes, "The Angels of Midnight's Eden, when approached in vain, or with a profane heart, shall ever manifest as enemies: The Garden is their sacred preserve, they are charged to stand guard over it lest it be abused. In so doing they will employ all powers at their command, including deception, delusion, confusion, torment, madness, disease, and death" (2005).

Which brings us to the second part of the answer to the question of whether the path of plant knowledge remains perilous in our times. Because our culture tends to view all non-ordinary states of consciousness and all communication with plants as deception, delusion, confusion, and madness, most people are not especially good at recognizing when the madness that is the curse of a disrespected plant shows up in the people around them, or even in themselves. But that does not mean that it is not a common occurrence. I have seen people who sought to claim the power of Datura as their own turned into grotesque versions of their misunderstandings of what power is. I have seen people who outsourced their spiritual work to Ayahuasca become glassier and more vacant and possessed of strange visions that do not seem to resonate with any world beyond their minds. I have seen Cannabis growers who put their obsession with money ahead of their love of the plant become prisoners of their own paranoia. (And lest you misunderstand, when treated with respect, I have seen all these medicines open the way to insight, liberation, and healing. But nothing can heal that cannot also harm. Those who wish to work with plants would do well to remember this. Just because our culture has forgotten taboos does not mean that the forces the taboos warned about have ceased to be active in the world.)

And being loved by other-than-human realms is not without peril either. The Scottish poet Thomas the Rhymer fell asleep beneath a Hawthorn and woke to find the queen of Elfland there, who showed him three roads he might travel—each road corresponding to another way of being in the world:

O see ye not that narrow road,
So thick beset with thorns and briers?
That is the path of righteousness,
Tho after it but few enquires.

The road to righteousness is the road laid out by the rules and laws of civilization—rules that bind instinct with tangled thorns and briers that threaten to cut all who would deviate from the path. It is marked by the logical consciousness that is centered in the brain—the consciousness that divides the world into categories that mark clear lines between what is right and true and acceptable and what is "beyond the pale." Its origins lie in the construction of the first walls that separated the city from the "wilderness"—the name people gave to the living world around them when they began to forget they drew their life from it. (The phrase "beyond the pale" itself derives from an English phrase describing the parts of Ireland that existed outside the original English zone of colonial control around Dublin in the late Middle Ages.)

And see not ye that braid, braid road,
That lies across that lily leven?
That is the path to wickedness,
Tho some call it the road to heaven.

The road of wickedness is the road of instinct uncoupled from any sense of consequence—a sense that arose organically when people experienced themselves as inextricably woven into webs of human and ecological connection. With disconnection came alienation, and with alienation came unassuageable hunger and insatiable lust that rip and tear at the fabric of being. The road appears broad and easy because all sense of limitation is lost; it appears to lead to heaven because it's the path of following unchecked desire, but it leads further and further from the source of being and life that offers the only true fulfillment of those desires.

Rather than bringing satiety, this path disconnects us from the heart, and it brings agitation that can grow into panic as people desperately seek pleasure to take the edge off their feeling of emptiness. And as each moment of pleasure fades, they find themselves feeling the emptiness more acutely and more frantically seek to stave off the gnawing feeling inside them. The true destination of this path is the realm of the hungry ghosts who have mouths but no stomachs and so eat and eat but are never full.

> And see not ye that bonny road,
> That winds about the fernie brae?
> That is the road to fair Elfland,
> Where thou and I this night maun gae.

The third road leading from the Hawthorn is the path of the heart. It's a path that leads to a wilder place, a place outside all ideas and judgments of right and wrong and good and evil, a place beyond and beneath and before the stories of guilt, fear, and shame we all carry. A place of wild innocence, where you can remember your connection to the world around you, and your desires arise from your response to its unspeakable beauty.

Hawthorn nourishes and calms the heart, helping to settle the *shen*. At the same time, her thorns offer protection from those who would harm you. Calm and protected, you can breathe into the center of your chest, opening to the core of your being.

Standing in that stillness and openness, the third road opens to you—leading you deep within, where you come into contact with the part of you that remains connected with All Things, where you can experience pure ecstasy.

Thomas followed that road and disappeared from civilization for seven years. He returned with the blessing and the curse of the "tongue that could not lie." He was no longer able to participate in the lies of politics and commerce that are necessary to operate within the framework of society. But he was also no longer able to lie to himself, no longer able to deny his own beauty and power. The luminosity of the Otherworld shone from his eyes. Its music flowed from his lips.

There are many techniques—dancing, drumming, and yogic practices among them—that can induce profound shifts in consciousness and can open us to a deeper awareness of other levels and dimensions of reality like the realm where Thomas spent his seven years.

Mind-altering preparations made from plants, fungi, and their synthetic analogs have played a role in most cultures' attempts to access other worlds. In most cases, the rites conducted with mind-altering plants were either rites of initiation occurring at times of major life changes or rites performed by shamans or priests on behalf of the community to seek insight and help from the spirit realm. In some cultures, the entire community would occasionally come together and use plant and fungal sacraments to access Otherworld guidance, but always within a ritual container. Occasionally, in some places, a person would take mind-altering medicines and go out into the wilderness alone to see wisdom, healing, insight, or transformation. But whatever the sacrament, whatever the culture, these medicines were always used with clear intent, grounded in a basic sense of the geography, ecology, and etiquette of the realm being accessed, as well as reverence for the spirits whose help was being asked. They were also always preceded and followed by ritual purification.

Yes, these rituals were sometimes joyous and celebratory—but those celebrations took place among people who had known each other all their lives and trusted each other deeply, something that is a rarity in the modern world. There have been times and places where people have succeeded in creating beautiful psychedelic celebrations in the modern world—I think of the way in which the Grateful Dead worked to weave together the consciousness of a crowd and let that collective mind find expression in and be guided by the music—but even the best of these modern large-scale events have their share of psychic casualties.

We live in a culture that emphasizes the right of individuals to go wherever they please and behave in whatever way suits them, which gives rise to the stereotype of the obnoxious, entitled American traveler that people hold in many parts of the world. Ours is also a culture that views the Otherworld we access when we work with mind-altering medicines as a mere dimension of the individual imagination. The pairing of these two attitudes and a lack of attention to the context in which we are engaging these medicines—the set and setting, to use the terms coined by Dr. Timothy Leary—can have dangerous consequences. I have spent long, harrowing nights in first-aid tents at festivals, taking care of people who became frightened, angry, agitated, and at times even violent and abusive when they let go the reins of their consciousness for the first time in a large crowd and discovered worlds of inner and outer darkness they were not prepared to navigate.

Yes, on one level, we should all have the freedom to explore our own consciousness and the ways it flows together with the mind of the living world—but with that freedom comes responsibility in all realms. With that caveat I want to speak of visionary medicines with some more specificity.

Cannabis is one of the oldest ritual medicines used by humans, and it has the effect of opening the senses both to the connections between things in this world and to the presence of the Otherworld. It makes our consciousness more permeable, for better or for worse. I often combine it with grounding, protective herbs like Wood Betony, Yarrow, and Mugwort to ward off baleful influences. When it opens the gates of sensation and perception too widely, and a person becomes foggy from sensory overwhelm, Holy Basil or Calamus can be helpful in clearing that fog.

European folk magic historically favored the use of visionary plants from the Nightshade family—plants like Henbane, Belladonna, and Datura—that require great caution, as the difference between a psychotropic dose and a fatal dose can be small. Traditionally they were infused in animal fat and given either orally or vaginally—the likely origin of the image of the witch riding a broomstick. These are complex medicines, but one of their primary influences is on the brain's mechanisms of assigning meanings to connections. Herein lies another dimension of their danger. When used with discernment, these medicines can help with perception of subtle patterns in the world, and they are useful aids to divination. When used recklessly, they can lead the mind to make connections that are not really there and then following these connections outward into madness. In addition to creating more physical casualties than other visionary medicines, the visionary Nightshades seem to create a lot more psychological and spiritual casualties. Habitual use can lead to joint pain similar to those experienced by people with Nightshade allergies.

Plants and fungi with chemical compounds similar to serotonin tend to facilitate greater connection with the living world. Serotonin flows and synaptic networks branch in fractal patterns that resemble the patterns in nature. (In fact, people who spend a long time in the wilderness alone experience significant spikes in serotonin levels that lead to a greater attunement to the subtle sensory information coming in from the world around them and a greater ability to think in nonlinear ways.)

Psilocybin flows and mycelial networks spread and intertwine with the roots of grasses that drink it in and begin to branch anew, growing deeper and more complex. It is only science's unscientific fear of anthropomorphism—the practice of seeing human structures and behaviors in other-than-human creatures—that stands in the way of many making the connections between the role tryptamines like serotonin and psilocybin play in facilitating human consciousness, the role they play in facilitating signaling and processing (dare we say "communication"?) in plant and fungal communities, and the ways in which ingesting botanical, fungal, and synthetic tryptamines alters human consciousness.

But, then, we haven't done a terribly good job of exploring the role of serotonin in our own brains to begin with. Most of us are used to thinking of serotonin as the compound whose relative scarcity is the mark of depression, and hence as a regulator of our moods. That is not entirely wrong, but the truth is more complex.

While low serotonin levels are associated with certain kinds of depression and slowing the breakdown or reuptake of serotonin does seemingly lift the moods of some who experience this kind of depression, the association in both cases is more in the realm of correlation than of causation. (In the case of double-blind human studies of selective serotonin reuptake inhibitors, the medications are barely more strongly associated with positive changes than the placebos.)

Elevated serotonin levels are also associated with dominance in male macaques and extroversion in human children on playgrounds, leading some in the business-coaching world to refer to serotonin as a "leadership chemical." A few things are important to note, however: One is that macaques increase serotonin production after they attain dominant positions, rather than before, suggesting a role of serotonin in maintaining that position rather than in obtaining it. Similarly, human serotonin levels rise in association with positive social interaction.

Thus, so far we know that in one set of situations—where people feel disconnected from others—serotonin levels are low, and in situations where macaques or people are managing complex social networks at a higher level than their peers, serotonin is relatively high. But there is another association with serotonin in humans as well that may shed further light on the nature of the molecule.

Autistic people and our first-degree relatives (parents, siblings, and children) have high levels of brain serotonin. Many Autistic people also seem to have a genetic predisposition toward the production of lower levels of monoamine-oxidase (MAO), the compound responsible for oxidizing and hence breaking down (or, more literally, burning up) serotonin. MAO-inhibiting plants are combined with tryptamine-rich plants in many cultures to allow the tryptamines to survive the liver, reach the brain, and reach levels at which they will alter consciousness, something that can sometimes also be achieved through using tryptamine-rich plants as a smoke or a snuff. The most famous MAO inhibiting plant is Syrian Rue (not a true Rue), which gave rise to the myth of the flying carpet because Persian rug-makers using the seeds as a dye experienced floating sensations and altered perceptions. Because MAO is also responsible for breaking down norepinephrine and tyramine, which raise blood pressure when they reach elevated levels, it is important to use great caution with them if your blood pressure runs high and to avoid them completely if you are on drugs the elevate the levels of any of your neurotransmitters—especially antidepressants and the stimulants commonly used to treat ADHD. Some tryptamines, like psilocybin, are more prone to survive the liver and digestive tract intact than others, like DMT. Their action will still be further potentiated by an MAO inhibitor, for better or worse.

Physiologically, Autism is marked by the nonlinear proliferation of synaptic networks—a fact that has led those who want to make Autistic people act more like everyone else begin administering drugs that "prune" the synapses of Autistic children. Recent research suggests that this neurobiological variation has its origin in genetic variations going back to the origins of humanity—and perhaps beyond—that increase neurogenesis (the proliferation of neural networks) in order to enhance cognition. The experience that arises from this physiological variation is marked by increased sensitivity to sensory stimuli, nonlinear and systems-oriented thinking, and unusual relationships to the use of language (which can include both linguistic precocity and the complete inability to use spoken language, even within the same person on the same day). It is worth noting that in Ireland, both linguistically precocious children and children who could not speak were often considered faerie changelings, beings from the Otherworld switched out for beings from this world. That trope tragically finds its modern expression in people speaking of Autism as a monster that has taken away a "real child" rather than as a natural variation in the neurobiology of our species.

This makes sense when we look at the fact that Autism is marked by high serotonin levels and possibly by lower MAO levels. Throughout human bodies, serotonin is associated with organ growth. And in plant and fungal bodies, tryptamines closely related to serotonin—such as psilocybin and the plant-rooting hormone auxin—are associated with the proliferation of mycelial and root networks that we now understand are among the primary organs through which plants and fungi exchange chemical and electromagnetic signals. We can understand more when we begin to think about the ways that exogenous tryptamines impact human brains.

The dose-dependent effects of exogenous tryptamines on human perception, cognition, and behavior shed further light on understanding serotonin. LSD-25, lysergic acid diethylamide, is a compound based on a derivative of a compound produced by the ergot fungus (the compound fungus that was likely used to prepare the ordeal poison used in the initiation into the Eleusinian Mysteries in ancient Greece). Relatively large doses of LSD administered in a therapeutic setting, modeled after the Peyote ceremonies of the Native American Church, showed tremendous effectiveness in the treatment of alcohol addiction in clinical trials in Saskatchewan in the 1950s. It wasn't that people immediately stopped craving alcohol, but rather that they were launched down paths of emotional and spiritual exploration that led to their addressing the conditions that gave rise to their addiction. One study subject went on to develop a twelve-step process for working through the issues he faced—and then went on to insist that that twelve-step process was the only proper way to address addiction and left out the initial step of having an experience that reoriented his sense of reality. I personally have seen the twelve steps be life-saving for people who come to twelve-step programs having already had a spiritual epiphany that moved their relationship with the divine from the realm of the abstract to the realm of the experiential—be it a psychedelic experience, a religious ceremony, a near-death experience, time in the wilderness, or a life event that transformed their world permanently. In people who haven't first had that "come to Jesus" or "come to Gaia" moment, I have sometimes seen the system's rigidity deepen shame and guilt around relapses and failures, accelerating the downward spiral associated with failing to maintain complete abstinence.

Other early work with the compound demonstrated that in a therapeutic setting, with a patient who was ready to engage deeply, LSD could bring about a lasting reorientation of a personal sense of reality that could aid in addressing unresolved traumas and in diminishing the anxiety and dread associated with death. Recent pilot studies have shown similar results with psilocybin in addressing Tobacco addiction and in helping patients with terminal illnesses engage the reality of their imminent deaths.

The introduction of psilocybin and LSD into a culture that lacked rituals for transforming consciousness resulted in both creative and destructive chaos—and, of course, the difference between the two is in the eye of the beholder. The nonlinear creativity that human encounters with exogenous tryptamines engendered in the minds of mathematicians, scientists, and engineers was tolerated as long as its sources were not talked about too openly and too loudly, and as long as its results could be harnessed and commodified. The cultural creativity that ensued was less welcome, especially when it amplified currents that were dissolving structures of obedience to social norms. And there were, of course, also psychedelic casualties—people whose unbounded opening of consciousness resulted in nonlinearly creative patterns that wrought harm on themselves and others and who had nobody capable of helping them integrate their experiences and reorient themselves. This created a cultural panic, and since pharmaceutical companies were not especially interested in defending a compound whose therapeutic use involved a small number of intense sessions, the panic resulted in the compounds being outlawed.

My introduction to exogenous tryptamine came mostly through the remnant of the counter-culture that persisted in pockets of rural New England in the early to mid-1990s, a generation before the current psychedelic renaissance. "Heroic" doses designed to (hopefully temporarily) dissolve the ego were the norm, and the intention was connection with a deeper level of reality, perception of the weft and weave of the fabric of time and space. I was a bit reckless and incredibly lucky.

Without any knowledge of Autism's neurobiology, I quickly came to intuitively understand that the difference between my brain on four or five hits of acid and my brain on a normal day was roughly equivalent to the difference between my brain on a normal day and someone else's brain without psychedelics. This meant and means that I was remarkably good at perceiving deep patterns in the world but that, even when sober, my skills at grocery shopping and balancing checkbooks were and are roughly equivalent to those of a tripping person. It also has an interesting effect on the nature of the relationships and connections I engage and experience.

One interesting role of serotonin and its analogs is their effect on how we experience empathy. Research into empathy in humans tends to suggest the existence of at least two varieties of empathy.

The variety most researched and discussed is cognitive empathy: the ability to correctly ascertain what another person is thinking and wanting and to respond in a socially appropriate way. The second, less researched and understood form of empathy is more somatic in its nature and, in some ways, is closer to the etymological implications of the word empathy—the ability to feel what someone else is feeling.

Our culture favors people whose cognitive empathy is strong and who are thus adept at navigating social situations, but who also have enough somatic empathy to be able to tune in—to some degree—to another person's experience intuitively and make small adjustments to the scripts they enact. These capacities seem to be associated with the "leadership" qualities seen in people with moderately high serotonin levels.

As somatic empathy increases above a certain threshold, cognitive empathy seems to decline (and vice versa). Autism is characterized by a high degree of somatic empathy—sometimes to a debilitating level, where other people's feelings become physically overwhelming for an Autistic person—and challenges with cognitive empathy that result either in breaches of social etiquette or in rigid adherence to learned and practiced social norms in a way disconnected from the experiences that give rise to them. Some kinds of trauma result in similar shifts.

Cognitive empathy also has an implied set of rules about who and what is deserving of our empathy. Somatic empathy knows no such rules. And hence Autistic people are also more likely to empathize with other-than-human beings than neurotypical people are. Sometimes we even feel empathy of what others perceive to be inanimate objects—be they mountains or computer operating systems.

Shifts in empathy that mirror the Autistic experience are common when people take large doses of exogenous tryptamines. And that seems to be part and parcel of their ceremonial role in many cultures: increasing the impulse for connection until it reaches a level that transcends family and community and reaches to the entire forest or the entire planet or the entire galaxy. For this reason, Gail Bradbrook, one of the founders of the Extinction Rebellion movement, has suggested that more people should take psychedelics with the intention of feeling their connection with the earth more deeply. In the proper ritual setting, I could see this being a collective initiation ritual for our times, but the ways in which to do that properly in this time and place are not yet clear.

Herein lies the danger to the dominant culture that tryptamine-bearing plants and fungi—and Autistic people—bring: the danger that if the perspectives they engender spread, then trees will cease to be lumber and people will cease to be "human resources" and our way of living will have to change. Which is precisely why tryptamines, human and wild, are such necessary molecules for our times—and precisely why they need to be engaged with caution and respect.

> *The magic power of a poem consists in it always being filled with* duende, *in its baptising all who gaze at it with dark water.*
>
> —*Federico García Lorca*

Mad, dead, or a poet
was never really
a choice:

once you have held
the Silver Branch
and gazed
into the abyss
that lies beneath
the dark waters
of the well
that feeds
the rivers
of the senses
and the rivers
of the world

you will
always
carry the
scent of the
Otherworld,

the obsidian
shimmer
of duende's
baptism
in dark water,

only poetry
can resolve
the torrents
into madness,

only poetry
can shape
the breath
to feed
the fire
that feeds
the forge
of the heart
that shapes
the spirit
like molten
iron

like the
molten iron
that rises up
from the
heart
of the earth
and sets
ablaze

the fire
at your root

and the fire
in your blood

and the fire
in your head

that blazes
in eyes

that shine
like the
Midsummer
Bonefire

and pours
forth from
the tongue

in words
that
bless

and words
that curse
and words
that command
roots
to break
through
sidewalks

and forests
to rise
where cities
now stand,

that like
the wind
in the desert
Ezekiel knew
commands
the dry bones
to live.

The fires
of a burning
world

have leapt
into my head,
and find
their match

in the
scarlet leaves
reflected
in the water

and the
red light
of Mars
in the sky.

In times
like this
my ancestors
donned feather cloaks

and went alone
into the forest

and ate autumn's
strange underworld fruit
that bloomed forth
after the rains,

spread across
the ground
like Hazelnuts,

holding
the memory
the forest
infused
into the topsoil,

and gazed
into the waters

until the fire
cooled enough

for the visions
to condense
and rain down

as words
sweet enough
upon the tongue

to soothe
the way
truth burns,

and returned
to the people

hoping to conjure
in their hearts
the rhythm
and in their breath
the song

that would
make the
wasteland bloom.

THIRTEEN PLANT ALLIES

What does it mean to call a plant an ally?

As a poet and a witch, I believe that words used with precision have great power to shape someone's experience of the world. The word *ally* comes from the Old French, *alier,* meaning "to join in marriage." Originally a verb, the word was first used as a noun in the fourteenth century to mean "kin."

It speaks of intimacy, tenderness, and trust. A deep knowing.

It begins with coming to know a plant on its own terms. Getting down on the ground and sitting with the plant. Coming back to it again and again. Coming to know the way the light shines on the plant at different times of day. The scent of the soil where it grows. The way the air tastes around the plant. Coming to know the body of the plant the way you would come to know the body of a lover. Knowing the feeling of its leaves and petals against your skin. Coming to love the ways it curves toward the sun.

And it requires getting quiet enough to notice what the plant stirs in you. The subtle sensations in your body. The memories, emotions, images, scents, and snatches of music that come to you. The ways your dreams change. Like a lover or a dear friend, a plant will teach you things you didn't know about yourself, new ways of being in your own body, new ways of being in the world.

Don't make the mistake of thinking that what you are learning and experiencing is all in your head. Don't think that to speak of a plant in the same terms you would use to describe a beloved is to lie and think and speak in metaphor. If you treat any of this as a metaphor, you will miss out on the chance to experience this other being in all of its magnificence—and to see your own beauty and power from the perspective of the plant.

But when coming to know a plant truly mirrors, in every way, the process of falling in love, everything changes. The idea of the world as sacred and alive opens into the experience of a world in which another consciousness embodied in a wildly different form from your own can speak directly to your heart.

The utilitarian view of the plant falls away. The answer to the question "What is Skunk Cabbage good for?" shifts from "Skunk Cabbage is good for calming spasms and clearing fluid from the lungs" to "Skunk Cabbage is good for setting roots deep in the mud, and melting its way through the ice to blossom forth in a gorgeous purple flower." Or "Skunk Cabbage is good for being Skunk Cabbage."

And the quality of the medicine and magic you work with the plant changes as well—the plant goes from being an inert substance chosen according to memorized sets of indications and properties and correspondences to being an active participant in shared work. New ways of working with the plant will emerge from your relationship.

And the relationship will demand of you consistency and honor. You will find yourself compelled to keep commitments you have made to spending time with the plant. And your respect for the plant will grow from an intellectual belief in the importance of avoiding overharvesting to a deep personal investment in seeing the plant flourish and defending the places it calls home.

This is not a path for the faint of heart. Like any intimate relationship, a true alliance with a plant will make you look at aspects of your life—patterns of thought and feeling and action—that you would rather ignore. And unbound by human etiquette, plants, like gods, will not change the subject or gloss things over with niceties and half-truths.

To deeply meet and be deeply met by a consciousness that exists so far outside the ideas and beliefs and stories and ideologies and hang-ups of our culture is to be seduced into wandering out through a gap in the crumbling wall around our civilization and into the borderlands where the lines carefully drawn and habitually held between humanness and wildness begin to dissolve. It is these borderlands where the greatest healing, the strongest magic, the deepest transformation occur.

I want to introduce you to thirteen of the allies I work with most frequently and most deeply. Your relationships with each of them will not be the same as mine, even if you apply their medicine in the same ways that I do, but I hope that my descriptions of the ways I work with each of them and of the nature of their medicine will be of use to you as you begin to develop your own plant relationships.

Lobelia *(Lobelia inflata)*

Lobelia is the quintessential herb for relaxing tension. Matthew Wood recently described it to me as the herb that awakens that autonomic nervous system and hence the Animal Self. I think of it is as the key that unlocks the cage that tension has created to contain the Animal Self. This means, of course, you have to be somewhat careful with it, because sometimes a caged animal runs for the forest when set free, but sometimes that caged animal responds with fear and rage that had been pent up during the time of its imprisonment. It first entered the pharmacopeia of the English-speaking world through the work of the cantankerous New Hampshire farmer and herbalist Samuel Thomson in the early years of the current republic. Thomson used it to clear the way for the fire of the body to burn away illness.

Most people, on taking Lobelia, feel an irritation in the back of their throat—this is the stimulation of the acrid taste receptors, resetting the signal the vagus nerve is carrying through our body, restoring channels of communication between the major centers of our nervous system (the brain, the heart, the gut, and the genitals), reaffirming safety, inviting us to enter an open and relaxed state.

This is followed by the action of the alkaloid lobeline on receptors. It further encourages the release of tension without sedating awareness, an action similar to the action of nicotine in the body. This alkaloid also works synergistically with acetylcholine to help consolidate learning and memory—nicotine does the same thing, but with nicotine, there is damage to the receptor sites for acetylcholine, which can lead, over time, to cognitive decline. With Lobelia there is no such damage. Lobeline also helps the body slow the conversion of dopamine—which is involved in the creation of motivation, reward, and meaning—to norepinephrine, which narrows the focus and creates anxiety when its levels are too high. For this reason, I use the herb not only with anxious people but also with people whose flat depression follows a period of intense stress that led to a depletion of dopamine. In these instances I like to combine it with high doses of the dopaminergic herb Brahmi *(Bacopa monnieri)* and a little bit of an MAO inhibitor like Puncture Vine *(Tribulus terrestris)* or, if it is available, Syrian Rue *(Peganum harmala)*. I will omit the MAO inhibitor if the person is taking antidepressants or if their blood pressure tends to run high.

Take a moment to think about the places where you see people smoking Tobacco most frequently: outside veterans' halls, twelve-step meetings, and emergency rooms. In war zones and prisons. In bus stations and back alleys. People smoke Tobacco in these situations because they need to release tension without losing their focus on their surroundings. Most people in these same situations will benefit from Lobelia.

The second thing most people experience when they take Lobelia is an expansion of the airways, a relaxation and opening of the chest, and a softening of the diaphragm. This allows the breath and the heart rate to normalize, helping someone become more present in their body. The sense of opening it brings to the chest is similar to that brought by stimulating the Pericardium 6 (PC 6, Nei Guan: Inner Gate) acupuncture point, which lies three finger widths down from the scaphoid between the tendons of the wrist. The pericardium, in Chinese medicine, is the heart protector, and both drop doses of Lobelia and stimulation of PC 6 help to reopen someone's awareness to what is present here and now. I've had particularly good results applying a drop of Lobelia directly to that acupuncture point. The physical pericardium, which holds and supports the physical heart, rests only when the heart is supported by the diaphragm during the brief pause we take between inhalation and exhalation. I experience particularly strong opening up of the breath and of awareness when, while applying Lobelia to PC 6, I also lengthen the pause between inhalation and exhalation. I suspect the combination is helping to restore heart rate variability.

Lobelia is also an herb I use in emergency situations to open the airways. The flowers of the species were considered "official" in the pharmacopeia until it was deemed "too capricious" and removed from use in conventional medicine. *Lobelia inflata* has flowers whose form resembles the air sacs in the lung. Some herbalists favor *Ephedra* species, an emergency bronchodilator, but *Ephedra* and its eponymous alkaloid, ephedrine, open the airways by stimulating the sympathetic nervous system response, inducing anxiety.

Lobelia is often one of the first herbs that I will give someone, because it brings them into a clear, grounded presence that opens the way for other medicines to move through the body. Most formulae I make have at least a little bit of Lobelia for that purpose.

I have also worked with Lobelia ritually in situations where constrictions and restrictions block the path forward. My simplest way of working with any plant magically is to take a drop of a tincture, a sip of tea, or a puff of smoke into my body and ask the plant spirit to instruct me in ways of dealing with the situation at hand.

Vervain *(Verbena* spp.*)*

Both the American and the European species of Vervain are tremendously helpful in releasing tension when the sources of the tension is the person's own intense drive to meet the impossibly high standards they set for themselves.

Matthew Wood writes that Dr. Edward Bach brought out the "genius of the plant. . . 'The typical Vervain patient,' says Dr. Bach, 'has an intense attitude towards life. He or she is strong-willed, enthusiastic, generally not able to relax. This drives the person to overexertion, both mental and physical. They refuse to be beaten and will carry on long after others would have given in. They have found fixed ideas and are very certain they know that they are right. They may be obstinate in refusing treatment until compelled. Then they may be carried away by their enthusiasm and cause themselves much strain'" (2009).

Wood also taught me that people who benefit from Vervain tend to hold tension in the back of their necks and are usually compulsive list-makers. When people hear this profile, they often think of ruthless type A business executives. But Vervain is also the herb of the activists who sacrifice their health out of dedication to justice and liberation, the social workers and teachers and public defenders who take their work home with them and go above and beyond anyone's most stringent expectations to help people struggling to survive. It is the herb for the immigrants who travel across deserts and flooded rivers and face official and unofficial armed forces in order to finally be able to get to the United States or Canada, where they will work seventy hours a week for less than minimum wage and send almost all their money back to their family in Mexico or Honduras or Nicaragua or El Salvador. It is the herb for the parents of chronically ill children who train themselves in medicine and law and the navigation of bureaucracy so they can fight better and harder for their children's health. Even though what all of these people are dedicated to is utterly necessary, they still need help in relaxing their intense drive. They need to be able to pace themselves for the long haul. And when I give them Vervain, I tell them exactly that. They often need to be reminded the necessity of health and rest and restorative pleasure in sustaining their body, so they can continue doing the work they give themselves to so completely.

One interesting thing about tension in the back of the neck is that it prevents a person from refocusing awareness deeper in the body by restricting the flow of blood and cerebrospinal fluid. More blood concentrates in the head, where the mind's ideas of how things should be are separated from the visceral experience of how things are. Without access to new sensory and emotional information, the Human Self goes into overdrive, trying to come up with solutions to the problems it perceives, and pursuing those solutions with greater and greater urgency.

Matthew Wood makes the connection between the people Vervain helps most and the "stiff-necked people" the Bible refers to—those whose personal will and desires prevented them from receiving and listening to wisdom. This connection recently helped me understand the role the European Vervain, *Verbena officinalis*, played for Gaulish druids, who used it to prepare people to receive visions.

I had long been puzzled by the idea of Vervain as a visionary plant, because even *Verbena officinalis*—which Wood says works at a deeper spiritual level than the North American *Verbena hastata*—doesn't induce the immediate kind of visionary shift I associate with herbs typically used to connect with the Otherworld. But in order to open the way for vision, it is necessary to be able to descend into an open and receptive state, and Vervain can help prepare the way. Vervain is also spoken of as an ancient herb of purification, and here I think of the ways that tension held in the neck is often the result of internalizing expectations, and releasing that tension releases those influences.

Wood also points to an interesting signature of the European variety of Vervain: its flowering tops evoke the image of the antlers of the Stag. He says that people feel that influence most strongly in places where that traditional association exists, even if they are not fully aware of the strength of that historical connection.

Vervain played a significant role as an herb of protection and purification in the Irish tradition. Bitter plants are often plants of protection, because they help to ground us more fully in our bodies, making it harder for us to succumb to outside influences. The only major European herb of protection I am aware of that is *not* bitter is St. John's Wort—but St. John's Wort does strengthen and stimulate the part of the nervous system associated with the solar plexus, and it stimulates the liver to purify the blood in the same way that bitter plants do.

Both Vervain and St. John's Wort are among the seven herbs that folklorist Niall Mac Coitir says cannot be harmed by anything natural or supernatural if harvested properly (2017). The same seven herbs were also used for cursing if collected at night on Bealtaine while invoking a baleful power. This is consistent with the traditional concept that power drawn from the Otherworld is morally neutral and is given valence by the intentions of those who wield it.

Lady Jane Francesca Wilde—who was one of the earliest scholars to make the connection between remnant Pagan practices in Ireland and the religion of Neolithic Indo-European migrants whose Indian ancestors' customs and practices also gave rise to the Hindu religion—gives this account of Vervain's ritual use in her native County Wexford in the late nineteenth century: "The Hindus had their cattle, or cow festival in spring, when they walked round the animals with great ceremony, always going westward, while they flung garlands on their horns. So in Ireland there was also a procession, when the cows were decorated with vervain and the rowan, and were sprinkled with the *Sgaith-an-Tobar* (the purity of the well), that is, the first water drawn from a sacred well after midnight on May Eve."

Mac Coitir recounts a similar practice in Kilkenny, where farmers walked the boundary of the land, sprinkling it with water taken from a holy well on May Eve and then blessing their Cattle in the same way. This connects the plant directly with the blessings of the Otherworld.

And if you are feeling too overwrought to access those blessings, Vervain will help you come to the place of being able to relax and allow them to come in.

Agrimony *(Agrimonia eupatoria)*

Agrimony is a plant I like to share with people whose tension is the result of being unable to express important truths or important aspects of who they are, because they would face heavy consequences if they spoke freely. It's the medicine I give them after they have safely extricated themselves from the situation they were stuck in. Matthew Wood explains this:

> *The characteristic mental state of the Agrimonia patient revolves around tension, frustration, anger, and inner torment. The person feels "caught in a bind," as if he or she is in the wrong place at the wrong time, unable to do the right thing, go with the flow, or be a good person. Often the problems revolve around the work situation. The person is in the wrong job for his or her interests and talents or working for a frustrating employer or supervisor. This mental tension builds to such proportions that the person feels tortured. Instead of manifesting this tension outwardly, what is highly typical of the Agrimonia patient is the effort to hide the true feelings beneath a façade.*

Often that façade is a tortured smile, but I have also often seen people who hide their anger and pain beneath expressions of equanimity benefit from Agrimony.

Being "caught in a bind" also describes the experience of enduring oppression. Oppressed and marginalized people deal with constant sleights and insults to fundamental aspects of their being—and often find themselves hiding behind a façade in the face of these microaggressions and macroaggressions in order to avoid even greater harassment, punishment, or violence. The trans person who is consistently and deliberately called by the wrong name and wrong pronouns by their boss, the Black man repeatedly stopped by police when driving in his own neighborhood, and the woman constantly subjected to misogynist "jokes" on construction sites are forced to stifle their authentic responses to these assaults on their dignity or face tremendous repercussions. Agrimony might be a remedy for each of these people. When I treat people in these kinds of categories, the conversation I have with them about Agrimony is especially important.

Agrimony releases the tension that is holding back the anger. That is a good thing. But it needs to happen in the right setting and in the right way. If the person is caught in a fundamentally unsafe situation, the wrong release of that anger could have devastating consequences. Even if the person is in a relatively safe situation, Agrimony might still release flashes of anger and sharpness that could damage relationships. So when I am giving someone Agrimony, I always talk with them about the anger that it might release and work with them to develop a way to safely and intentionally move and release and express the anger. Many people seem to really like smashing old dishes. Personally, I use weightlifting to complete the release of what is moving through my body.

The tension can also be holding back pain. Matthew Wood taught me that the person who benefits from Agrimony will often hold their breath in the face of intense pain or emotion. This helps to dull the intensity of the sensation, but it does not allow the emotion to move through the body. Agrimony, especially in combination with Lobelia, releases the tension in the diaphragm that is preventing breath—and emotion and sensation—from moving freely.

Agrimony isn't effective only when we are actively caught in an external situation where our truth is restrained, it also helps with releasing the constriction caused by internalized oppression. We hold ourselves back by accepting degrading stories about us in order to protect ourselves from coming into contact with oppressive forces outside us, and then we begin habitually suppressing our authentic expression, because we see it as unacceptable. Draja Mickaharic writes, "Agrimony is used to break the most common curses, those which you impose on yourself through fear and guilt" (2020). Such curses often break in storms of grief and rage followed by a surge of vitality.

Black Cohosh *(Cimicifuga racemosa)*

Black Cohosh is a plant with dark, gnarled, twisted roots that give rise to a tall stalk topped with a spray of white flowers. It is native to Appalachia and is threatened by overharvesting in its native habitat, so please seek Black Cohosh from growers who cultivate it, or, better yet, if you live somewhere where it will thrive, grow it yourself.

Black Cohosh is indicated when someone is in despair, brooding over loss and pain and worry, with grief hanging over them like the proverbial black cloud. There is often tension and dull ache in the trapezius, a hunched-over posture, and a heavy feeling in the chest. These people will also have a tendency to take on other people's grief.

I think of the spray of white flowers, high above the gnarled root, as the stars that show the way up out of the abyss—or at least bring the reminder that there is a world beyond the well. The well of grief can be an important place to spend time. In Irish tradition, all the rivers and streams of the world have their root in a well in the Otherworld beneath our feet—the place of all beginnings and endings. To me, the well of deep grief is that same well, and, awash in its waters, we release the meanings the world held before and prepare ourselves to create new meaning as we relate to the world in a new way. But eventually we need to return to the world. And I have found Black Cohosh helps to shift the stagnant emotions that are weighing me down and help me see the starry sky. This reminds me that the iron in my blood and the iron at the core of the earth were forged together in the first generation of stars, that I am connected with everything.

Many contemporary herbalists speak of Black Cohosh as working on estrogen levels through various proposed mechanisms that shift and change as each model becomes outdated. They presume that the depression Black Cohosh treats is associated with estrogen levels, pointing to the greater prevalence of this kind of brooding depression before menstruation, the role of Black Cohosh in easing menstrual pain and in bringing on delayed menstruation, and anecdotal evidence that this kind of depression is most common in women. But I have used Black Cohosh to ease this kind of depression in people of all genders and with all kinds of hormonal profiles. If brooding depression is most prevalent among women, it may be because our society asks women to take on the responsibility for other people's emotions—especially those of men. And Black Cohosh's role in bringing on menstruation can be explained as much through its action on nerves, muscles, fascia, and fluids as it can by a hormonal model of its action.

The great nineteenth-century physiomedicalist physician William Cook saw Black Cohosh acting primarily on nerves and the serous tissues (fascia). Cook began his description of the plant's properties by writing: "The root of cimicifuga has long been known to American physicians as a remedy of decided and peculiar value; yet its true action has been enshrouded in so much uncertainty that the proper places to employ it have not been well defined. After much experience and careful observation in its use, I offer the following account of it, which I believe to be correct, though in many respects different from the descriptions usually given" (1869a).

Those words are equally apt today. Black Cohosh tends to be pigeonholed as a women's herb, a menopause herb, or a childbirth herb when, in fact, these specific uses are just extensions of the plant's broader capacity to work with the nervous system (and by extension, the muscles) to restore fluidity to experience.

Cook writes, "Its power is expended chiefly upon the nervous structures, beginning at the peripheries and extending to the brain, including the ganglionic system; through the sensory nerves influencing the heart and pulse, and through the sympathetic nerves making a decided impression upon the uterus. . . . On the nerves it acts gradually, yet in the end with decided power—soothing them, relieving pain dependent on local irritation, and proving a good antispasmodic."

A well-made Black Cohosh tincture has an earthy taste, like clean soil, with a hint of bitterness—it grounds us in the body. It has a hit of acridity, and the activation of the acrid taste receptor at the back of the throat sends a strong signal across the ventral branch of the vagus nerve, restoring coherent communication between the body's major centers of neurological activity and consciousness (the brain, the heart, the gut, and the genitals) and engaging the parasympathetic nervous system to relax muscular tension throughout the body.

Grounding in the body and improving the flow of communication between our major centers of consciousness makes Black Cohosh an ideal herb for bringing a person into calm, centered, embodied presence. It is through the heart that we take in the information that forms our emotional felt sense of the world. And it is through the ways in which the enteric portion of our autonomic nervous system reads the signals of tension and flow across the fascia that we gain our visceral sense of the experience of body and world in this location in time and space. Because of this, bringing these centers back into alignment and coherence fundamentally shifts our experience of embodiment. I think of Black Cohosh as realigning a vertical axis of embodied consciousness that also becomes our own *axis mundi*—the axis on which our own world turns. We can extend our awareness along that axis all the way down into the core of the earth, where we can anchor and reorient ourselves and remember who we are.

From this state, we are better able to address and process the grief and pain and fear held in the body. Here, too, Cook's insights guide us to seeing how Black Cohosh can restore the body to healthy flow: "On serous tissues it allays irritation, soothes excitement, and relieves sub-acute and chronic inflammation."

We can gloss the nineteenth-century use of the term *serous* tissue to refer to what Ida Rolf would call the fascia and stodgy anatomists would call the connective tissues, interstitia, and adipose tissues. The fascia hold our bodies' memories of tension and motion, and especially of patterns we have been unable to release. Osteopath Paolo Tozzi discusses this (2014):

Memories in the body may be also encoded into the structure of fascia itself. Collagen is deposited along the lines of tension imposed or expressed in connective tissues at both molecular and macroscopic level. Mechanical forces acting upon the internal and/or external environment, such as in postures, movements, and strains, dictate the sites where collagen is deposited. Thus, a "tensional memory" is created in a particular connective tissue architecture formed by oriented collagen fibers. This architecture changes accordingly to modification of habitual lines of tension, providing a possible "medium term memory" of the forces imposed on the organism. However, this type of signaling may be altered in pathological conditions. . . . The release of substance P from nerve endings, particularly driven by the hypothalamus following emotional trauma, may alter the collagen structure into a specific hexagonal shape, referred as "emotional scar." The entirety of this phenomenon may be interpreted as a highly structurally and functionally specific process of encoding memory traces in fascia.

Our bodies are mostly water, and the fluids flowing through the collagen bundles of our fascia are a medium of consciousness—carrying hormones and conducting electricity and light, including the biophotons produced by the DNA in the nucleus of every cell. The tissues they flow through are like layers of soil, holding the memory of emotion and sensation—and just as water absorbs the substances contained in layers of soil, so too those inner waters take on the chemical reminders and electromagnetic patterns of the past experiences encoded in the collagen structures.

Dancer and occult publisher Alkistis Dimech writes, "The matrix of connective tissue is the repository of our individual and ancestral memory. (cf. Freud's notion of an 'archaic heritage' and Jung's description of archetypes as 'biological instinctual constellations.') It is attuned to motion and emotion, which it registers and retains, submerged in and holographically distributed throughout the liquid crystalline continuum. This body memory, which is always oriented to the future—that is, to survival and evolution—is engaged directly through the dynamics of the living body."

Where the body holds patterns of tension and constriction, tissues tend toward low-grade inflammation (creating the dull aches for which Black Cohosh is specific). This creates swelling that further obstructs the flow of fluids, and emotions stagnate—contributing to the kind of dark, heavy, stagnant, brooding emotional state that Black Cohosh is also specific for. My best guess is that Black Cohosh brings down the inflammation in the tissues, allowing the fluids to flow again.

Time and time again I have watched Black Cohosh bring sensory and emotional memories to the surface to be processed and released in ways similar to deep body work. The difference I observe is that Black Cohosh's soothing action on the nervous system usually prevents the surfacing sensations and emotions from becoming too much for the person to bear.

I frequently combine Black Cohosh with Solomon's Seal *(Polygonatum biflorum)* or Shatavari *(Asparagus racemosus)*, which lubricate the fascia by promoting the secretion of synovial fluid—and which also make life juicier. Solomon's Seal is threatened in the wild, so please only buy from cultivated sources or grow your own. I will often also bring in a warming aromatic herb to encourage blood flow into—and out of—the tissues, because where blood flows, awareness goes and can shift. Which plant I will use will depend on some of the more esoteric qualities of the plants: I will use Calamus *(Acorus calamus)* if a person needs to bring their emotions and experience into expression, Wormwood *(Artemisia absinthium)* if the person has been beaten down by oppression and feels like the walking dead, Devil's Club *(Oplopanax horridus)* when a person needs to reassert their sense of self and their right to be alive and embodied in the world, and, if things feel physically cold and stuck, Ginger *(Zingiber officinale)*—an idea that comes from a formula Margi Flint once taught me for joint pain—Black Cohosh, Solomon's Seal, and Ginger—which was my introduction to the energetic pattern underlying all these combinations. Together, these herbs restore flow.

Black Cohosh eases the way for life to flow through us—and guides us toward the stars that were the furnaces that forged the elements of our bodies. It is a profound medicine for bringing people into embodied presence.

Wormwood *(Artemisia absinthium)*

Wormwood is a potent herb that helps to reawaken our memory of who we are. Modern conceptions of the herb tend to revolve around its use in treating parasitic infections—from malaria to pinworms—but physical parasites are not the only kind of "pernicious external influence" (to borrow a term from Chinese medicine) that Wormwood can help us drive out.

Our contemporary culture is one of the few that does not speak of possession as a source of illness. If we understand possession to mean the invasion of our own being by another consciousness that doesn't have our best interest in mind, a parasite of consciousness, and if we realize that such a being doesn't have to have a human-like form, we can see how we all give over a degree of mental and emotional control to disembodied forces. Is there a real difference between writing a document that gives a thought-form and a name to a corporation or a government and performing incantations and drawing sigils to summon angels and demons—especially when people then make decisions that prioritize the needs and desires and survival of that entity over their own values and well-being in exchange for money or protection? I would contend that as a culture, we do not speak of possession not because it is rare but because it is ubiquitous.

The late Dale Pendell contended that the Wormwood's old Saxon name, *wermod,* from which the word *vermouth* is also derived, meant "defend the mind" (2010). He was likely drawing on the work of an early twentieth-century philologist, Ernest Weekley, who theorized that *wermod* was a compound word whose components meant "man" and "courage."

The great seventeenth-century herbalist and astrologer Nicholas Culpeper said that his understanding and description of Wormwood contained the key to understanding his entire approach to medicine. Because of its profound heat and its tendency to grow near forges, Culpeper ascribed Wormwood's rulership to Mars and asserted that, in relation to humanity, Mars's "only desire is [that] they should know themselves."

In the Greek-derived medicine that Culpeper studied and practiced, heat is identified with the life force and cold is seen as breaking down a being's identity. The profound heat of Wormwood helps in reasserting that identity.

A generation earlier, Shakespeare seems to have tapped into this same aspect of Wormwood's medicine when he describes the faerie King Oberon using the herb, which he calls "Dian's bud" to break the spell he had cast on his queen, Titania, that caused her to fall in love with an ass. Giving the remedy, Oberon said:

Be as thou wast wont to be
See as thou wast wont to see:
Dian's bud o'er Cupid's flower
Hath such force and blessed power.
Now, my Titania, wake you, my sweet queen.

It is worth noting here that Matthew Wood says that Wormwood is an herb for someone who "wakes in a convulsion or a trance"—its heat stimulates the nervous system to rouse consciousness. Drawing on that usage, I frequently give drop doses of this herb to people experiencing intense nightmares and to people experiencing dissociation. In the latter case, I like to combine it with Calamus. In both cases, I combine it with Wood Betony *(Stachys betonica)*, an herb that helps people anchor more deeply in their bodies in the present time and space.

There is some interesting cultural blending at play here that suggests some ancient truths. The character of Titania is clearly based on the cultural memory of Celtic faerie queens, not yet tamed and diminished in the collective imagination as they would be in the Victorian Era, who embodied the spirit of the living land. Her name, however, is believed to be a variation on that of Diana, Roman goddess of the moon and the hunt, who, in turn, was a syncretized version of the Greek Artemis, who, like Pan, arose from the trace of the memory of wild spirits who people had known since the Paleolithic. Artemis gives her name to *Artemisia*, the genus of plants to which Wormwood belongs (which Shakespeare references by naming it "Dian's bud"). So, the medicine that cures Titania of her delusion and amnesia is, in fact, an herb that embodies her essence.

Titania, is, of course, portrayed as lusty and free, while Artemis and Diana are traditionally viewed as virginal. There is not, however, as strong a disconnect here as one might think at first. As German religious scholar

Julia Iwersen writes (n.d.): "The Greek Artemis is clearly the heiress of the Mistress of the Animals, but her wildness was acceptable in a patriarchal culture only if it was understood that she was not like other women. Thus she was superficially bereft of her female sexuality."

Of course, in a classical Athenian cultural framework, that "female sexuality" would have been understood as something that needed to be controlled and harnessed for the purposes of reproduction. Susun Weed and others have suggested that in such a context, "virginity" can be understood to mean being outside masculine control rather than necessarily implying chastity.

Certainly, this is the sense that I get from my own encounters with Artemis and her herbs. At one level, we can understand Wormwood and its cousin, Mugwort (which Culpeper saw as ruled by Venus), as herbs of the wild feminine outside of masculine control. On another level, as herbs that replace externally imposed concepts of identity with the identity that arises organically from within, they tend to break down our cultural categories of gender, and they frequently show up to help when I am working with people who in one way or another are struggling with the cultural and social constraints connected with the gender they were assigned at birth. Every time I work with any of the plants associated with Artemis, I hear a voice saying, "my gender is not feminine, it is wild."

This points to another important aspect of Wormwood's medicine. Matthew Wood writes that Wormwood "is suited to people who have been brutalized by the reverses of life, including poverty and abuse," especially when they are dealing with "chronic depression, lack of affect, deadness, hopelessness" (2008). In other words, it is an herb that is helpful when oppression causes depression by suppressing someone's sense of self and power.

I learned from Wood to give just one or two drops of Wormwood a week when someone is in that kind of flat, lifeless depression, because he warns that more than that can bring on further depression. My own sense here is that a tiny bit of Wormwood reawakens consciousness, but more of it brings suppressed things to consciousness.

When I am working with someone who is feeling grey and lifeless, I give one drop of Wormwood a week and work with drop doses of Angelica or Damiana in between those treatments.

I will give Wormwood more frequently when a person is actively working to reintegrate buried aspects of their consciousness, and in those cases, I give it in combination with Black Cohosh and Solomon's Seal or Shatavari. This combination is also indicated for the frequently co-occurring stiffness and rheumatic pain that arise from long-term body armoring.

Curiously, at highly concentrated doses, when distilled with other herbs to make absinthe, Wormwood has a somewhat opposite effect: it brings a fluid bliss to the body and changes the perception of light, giving it a shimmering, fluid quality as well. True absinthe is sadly illegal to sell in the United States because of concerns about its liver toxicity—which are largely based on old French propaganda about the drink. Absinthe was historically the drink of choice of bohemians and war veterans in France, two groups of people who drank heavily and acted strangely, and many of whom developed liver disease. Thujone, the major psychotropic compound in Wormwood (as in Yarrow and Mugwort and Cedar) can, indeed, be toxic to the liver. But in recent years, medical historians have concluded that those who died from drinking too much absinthe most likely died not of thujone poisoning but of alcohol-induced liver damage, though likely the combination of the two at large quantities with great frequency made them die somewhat faster than other alcohol addicts. However, there is little justification for the idea that absinthe is harmful in moderation.

The first time I had absinthe was the only time I (briefly) met Dale Pendell. He was teaching a workshop about absinthe and passed out samples during class. After the class, I was waiting in line to ask him a question, and the pitcher and paper cups came up and down the long line many times, and I partook each time. The workshop was on a beautifully landscaped college campus, and when I left the building, I found myself standing on a little wooden bridge over a pond with Water Lilies. As I looked at the water, it shimmered with exactly the quality of light Monet portrayed in his famous painting of a similar scene. It dawned on me that Wormwood taught Monet, who loved absinthe, that way of seeing light.

A few years later, a friend shared some beautiful absinthe with me during a conference in Alberta in late summer. When I walked outside a little while later, I saw the aurora borealis, a curtain of green light across the sky that was exactly the same color as the absinthe: the uncannily iridescent hue that gives absinthe the name *la fée verte*—the green fairie.

This dual nature of Wormwood: the ability to bring someone back more fully into this world or to help someone access a way of seeing more like that of the Otherworld is a quality it shares with its cousin Mugwort *(Artemisia vulgaris)*. (It is called Mugwort because of its popularity as an herb in beer before the laws replacing it with Hops spoiled everyone's fun.) Mugwort is famous as an herb for vivid dreaming, but I learned from Matthew Wood that it can also be an herb for helping someone who is too much in the Otherworld be more grounded in this one. I have found it especially helpful for artists, writers, and musicians who find that Cannabis inspires them to see things in new ways and gets their ideas flowing but also limits their follow-through in actually creating new work. I have them mix a bit of Mugwort with their Cannabis, and all report excellent results.

Damiana *(Turnera diffusa)*

Damiana is a light at the southwestern horizon reminding us that though the night descending is dark, morning will come. Bitter, warming, and aromatic, Damiana grounds us into our bodies, stirs our heart to quicken the rhythm of the movement of our blood, gently opens the airways, and relaxes the tension we hold to allow the blood to flow freely to all of our parts—and where blood flows, awareness goes.

In winters of snow and ice, winters of the heart, and winters of our collective experience, Damiana awakens the memory of the invincible summer within us that Albert Camus spoke of finding in the depths of winter. Damiana is well known for its capacity to stimulate pelvic circulation, bringing blood and awareness flowing to the genitals, giving rise to its reputation as an aphrodisiac. And it excels in this manner.

But to fully appreciate the stirring Damiana brings to the body, we need to broaden our definition of the erotic. Eros is the force that sets matter dancing, the embodied flow of life. By relaxing tension and increasing blood flow and sensation, Damiana invites us to inhabit our bodies more deeply, engaging eros in new ways. It is an herb of joyful embodiment, restoring sensual pleasure in all of its forms—dancing, touching, savoring delicious food, breathing in the scent of snow and Fir and Pine and woodsmoke.

I often give Damiana to elders who are living in a world that forgets that bodies of all ages need and desire sensual pleasure and to people recovering from injuries and illnesses who are learning to be in their bodies again. I sometimes combine Damiana with the Chinese herb *Corydalis yanhusuo*, usually used to diminish the intensity of pain signals to keep the return of sensation from being too overwhelming at first. Damiana is also delicious in honey and amazing in mead.

Like all bitter, warming, aromatic herbs, Damiana is a carminative, stimulating sluggish digestion and relieving gas and bloating. The latter action of carminatives is an important consideration in the timing of the administration of Damiana as an aphrodisiac in the conventional sense.

Hawthorn *(Crataegus* spp.*)*

Hawthorn calms and strengthens the heart and cools fires that burn too intensely in our blood vessels.

The heart moves out of balance, into excess, when our bodies and minds become overwhelmed with too much to process. We become agitated, unsettled, irritable, and reactive as our minds struggle to make meaning of what is happening around us. Our minds often end up spinning their wheels because they are not grounded in the present time and space—and because the amount and intensity of the information about potential threats they are dealing with and sensory stimuli that need to be deciphered exceeds their capacity.

That excited state is essentially the state we experience when we have too much caffeine—an alkaloid whose ubiquitous presence in our world has its roots in early capitalism and the trade in Coffee, Tea, and Cacao from newly colonized lands. You can tell a lot about a culture by its drugs of choice. At moderate levels, caffeine makes people awake and focused. At higher doses, it makes many jittery and nervous. As the dose increases, caffeine increases the activity of norepinephrine—which makes us narrow our mental focus and increase our feelings of fear and aggression—and inhibits serotonin, thus closing off more sensory information from the body and the world around it and decreasing nonlinear creativity. One French philosopher, living at the dawn of capitalism, who was known for drinking over five dozen cups of coffee in a day, infamously concluded that his thoughts, the belief structures, and ideas of his Talking Self, were the primary confirmation of his existence. His ideas would define the emergence of a worldview that saw mind and body as separate and distinct entities and privileged rationality over emotion, intuition, and even empirical experience.

Like caffeine, fear and overwhelm trigger the increase of more and more norepinephrine, narrowing the scope of and increasing the feverish speed of mental activity. They also curtail our capacity to make connections and our desire to seek connection, increasing alienation, which, in turn, increases fear and overwhelm.

Sometimes unrestrained panic and unrestrained grief and unrestrained rage represent the same kind of revolution occurring within a person's being, their sensual and emotional Wild Self pushing against the rational structures imposed by the Talking Self and the demands enforced conformity imposes on our bodies. The upwelling of emotion breaks a person's fixed sense of reality open, creating the possibility of the return of the repressed and the transformation of a person's sense of being and meaning.

When it is not safe to simply release the barriers and allow "madness" to run its course, a safer and slower response is to work with gentle, subtly cooling and grounding herbs to take the edge off the intensity of someone's experience. This allows them to move more smoothly through the experience of letting mental and emotional heat move through them and allowing them to return to grounded presence.

We are coming to understand the heart as a complex organ of perception that picks up on the subtle electromagnetic shifts that signal changes in our bodies and in the bodies of the living things around us. The heart relays these messages via the vagus nerve to the amygdala and to the right frontal cortex of the brain, where they are interpreted as emotion. In other words, the heart is just what our ancestors thought it was, an organ that shapes our felt sense of the world. In some ways, we can see the heart, the amygdala, and the right frontal cortex as forming an axis that is the physiological location of that aspect of our Wild Selves that seeks pleasure in connection.

Hawthorn's medicine is cool and dark, like the rich soil of an Apple orchard. It soothes the heart that is overheating from taking in too much from the outside world. What is too much? More than a person's amygdala and right frontal cortex can process. What situations will overwhelm a person vary widely, depending on how wide the sensory gates that allow information to pass from the heart to the brain are open, what associations they have with the sensations they are experiencing, and how much unprocessed emotion is held inside their body.

I love to tincture the leaf, flower, and berry together in a good Irish whiskey with a touch of honey—and include a single thorn. I will mix a little of the tincture with heavy cream when making offerings to the tree, my Irish ancestors, or the Daoine Sidhe.

I learned from Matthew Wood that Hawthorn is specific for reducing "heat and irritation in the capillaries." This explains the medicine's well-known ability to mitigate cardiovascular disease and also relates to its use in managing inflammation in the respiratory and digestive tracts—and its possible relevance in helping to manage the body's response to COVID-19 infection, as well as managing our responses to a world full of things that inflame our minds, our senses, and our tissues.

Hawthorn wasn't used for cardiovascular issues in the West until the early twentieth century, but it was widely used in medieval Europe to aid in the digestion of meat. Similarly, Hawthorn is used in Chinese medicine to treat indigestion.

In the 1990s, Dr. Deborah Frances pioneered the use of Hawthorn in the treatment of acute asthma attacks marked by "constriction and tightness in the chest." I've found it especially useful for asthma attacks brought on by emotional triggers and often preceded by heat in the cheeks and the ear lobes.

I am wary of making leaps from the conclusions of in vitro and animal studies of plant constituents to practical use of an herb with people, but when they line up with traditional knowledge of a plant and my own empirical experience, the three sets of evidence support and confirm each other. So it is with the research around Hawthorn and inflammation. I will just go into the basics here.

Hawthorn reduces inflammation in the epithelial cells of the lining of the respiratory tract and the walls of the blood vessels by preventing pro-inflammatory cytokines from recruiting white blood cells to the area. One Hawthorn constituent, vitexin, has been shown to act in a similar way to mediate inflammation in the respiratory tract.

Some polyphenols from Hawthorn also appear to inhibit ACE—angiotensin-converting enzyme, thereby weakening the action of angiotensin, a hormone that signals the body to constrict the blood vessels. Constricting blood vessels raises blood pressure and can also increase local inflammation by impeding healthy circulation. ACE converts raw angiotensin 1 into the active form of angiotensin, angiotensin 2. ACE has a counterpart, ACE2, which deactivates angiotensin 2, relaxing and opening the blood vessels.

This is particularly relevant now, because we are in the midst of a pandemic caused by a virus which dysregulates this particular system, a virus whose actions, I think, in many ways mirror and are exacerbated by our cultural tendency toward inflammatory responses to the world, both literal and figurative (which are ultimately one and the same—physiological inflammation brings inflammatory emotional responses, which create more stress, which creates more physiological inflammation). COVID-19 attaches itself to ACE2 receptors, initially in the lung, which interferes with the action of ACE2, thus increasing the action of angiotensin 2, causing blood vessels to constrict, spiking blood pressure, and causing tissue damage up to and including respiratory failure, scarring of the lung tissue, myocarditis, and kidney failure. Researchers are exploring whether flooding the body with ACE2 might be an effective way of treating COVID-19.

I don't know of any herbs that boost ACE2 levels, but in Hawthorn (and in Reishi), we have herbs that could theoretically help tilt the balance slightly in the right direction by inhibiting ACE and thus reducing levels of angiotensin 2 and somewhat reducing the need for ACE2. We also have other herbs that we know are vasodilators—like Black Cohosh, Yarrow, and Lobelia—that combine beautifully with Hawthorn. Vasodilating herbs have the added benefit of being diaphoretics, herbs that allow the body to disperse heat.

What happens with our breath effects our heart rate. What happens with the rhythm of the physical heart effects the emotional heart. This is not a metaphor. I work with Hawthorn when the outside world is overwhelming. Emotion and sensation build to a point when a person's internal processing becomes less and less coherent, and the body's inflammatory responses begin to kick in. Very often the person's ears will become hot and will even visibly redden just before the building heat triggers undirected explosive expression, a combined implosion and explosion where verbal communication becomes cut off but the body moves involuntarily with the force of the sensation moving through (which should never be forcibly stopped), or an inflammatory asthma attack.

Matthew Wood notes that Hawthorn is especially well suited for mental and emotional agitation in Autistic and other neurodivergent people, who, in Celtic cultures, would have been identified as faerie changelings, children from another world. He also notes that Hawthorn is heavily associated with the faerie realm in folklore. The Hawthorn, in fact, guards the gate between this world and the faerie world and so is well suited to those whose neurobiology's naturally resist the tight regulation of consciousness imposed by our culture. Hawthorn cools the heart and the blood to make us more receptive and less reactive to the world.

Calamus *(Acorus calamus)*

In Chinese medicine, the heart is the primary organ of consciousness and perception. The watery heart *yin* represents the heart's capacity to take in information from the world—it is nourished by beauty. The senses are spoken of as the "orifices of the heart." The fiery heart *yang* represents our capacity to express ourselves.

When we are overwhelmed with sensory and emotional information, the heart *yin* can overwhelm the heart *yang,* clouding the senses with a fog and first obscuring and then drowning out the fire of expression. Think of the heavy, dull feeling that lingers in your head after being in a noisy, crowded store with bright fluorescent lights in December.

Intense memories—sensation and emotion re-experienced outside their original context—bring their own fog, cutting us off from the experience of being present here and now. They can distort our perception of current events and prevent us from responding coherently.

Growing in the marshy muck of the shallows of lakes and ponds, Calamus, with its green rush-like leaves and its bright yellow flower, has a spicy root that clears the waters of the heart by reigniting the heart *yang.* Its sweet scent engages the senses, its bitterness grounds us and activates the enteric nervous system that processes the sensory information coming in from the fascia of the entire body, and its pungent heat focuses the mind and senses and stimulates circulation to the brain.

This makes it an especially important medicine for Autistic people like me. Sensory gating is the process by which people filter sensory information—including the felt sense of others' emotions and our own—so we only have to consciously interpret the information that is most important and most relevant, parameters set both by our belief structures and our bodies' past experiences. Autistic people tend to have wider open sensory gating channels than most people, which allows us to perceive things others miss but can also overwhelm us with information that we can have a hard time prioritizing and sorting. In response, we can go into sensory shutdown, and those of us who usually have access to speech can lose that access altogether.

When this happens to me, a few minutes in a dark room and a few drops of Calamus can often help me become reoriented and recover my ability to speak. Hawthorn is often a nice addition to the Calamus, helping to soothe the hyper-reactivity of my senses by cooling the heart (and possibly by reducing histamine and other pro-inflammatory compounds in my blood vessels). Schizandra can be a nice addition as well, helping to gather my attention inward toward my heart.

I associate Calamus with the Irish god Manannán Mac Lir, watery god of lakes and seas. Manannán gave his name to the Isle of Mann, where people climb the highest hill on the island with bundles of rushes on the Feast of John the Baptist, just after the summer solstice. The rushes growing in the marshes are "rent" for living on the land, paid to Manannán when the sun is at its brightest.

Though a god of wild waters, Manannán has a fiery nature in many ways, and perhaps because of the thundering sounds of the storm and the gentle music of wind and water that arise when he moves in this world, his magic is magic of vision, truth, and the word. When he is nourished by beauty and love, he sings. When his heart is wounded, his anguish is a tide none can withstand.

He bears a silver branch bedecked with golden apples from the Otherworld. Who holds the branch can see the world as he does, the world refracted through a teardrop. (His Beloved was named Fand Ní Aed Abra, meaning "tear who is the daughter of the fire of the eye." She was a goddess who helped to bring pleasure into the world.) The great ancient Irish King Cormac mac Art (Cormac, Son of the Bear) heard heavenly music when Manannán shook the branch. When Cormac himself saw it, he beheld the Otherworld Well wherein the Salmon of Wisdom dwells.

John Moriarty spoke of "Silver Branch perception," which sees the world as alive, and this world and the Otherworld as one Great World. This aligns with another capacity of Calamus—the capacity to refine perception and expression.

Ayurveda—which shares ancient cultural roots with Irish tradition going back to the Neolithic—speaks of kundalini, the vital force, likened to a rising serpent, that flows from its genital root up the spine to the head. (Ancient Greek and Middle Eastern traditions similarly spoke of twin serpents that climb the spine and are instruments of the fluid transmission of consciousness that leaves the body at death.) Ayurveda describes Calamus—which it calls Vacha, a Sanskrit word for "voice"—as an herb that purifies the kundalini to bring clear perception and understanding. It also has a long history of use in incense and anointing oils in Egypt and in much of the Middle East.

Calamus is not just an herb that aids in bringing forth speech—it aids in bringing forth the heart's purest truth. Herbalist jim mcdonald, who first introduced me to this herb, speaks of it as an herb that can help people when they plateau in their mental and emotional processing of their lives to achieve new insights, and I have seen Calamus do this again and again.

This is also an herb I give to people when they need the courage and clarity to speak difficult truths. If it had a motto, it might be that of the late Maggie Kuhn, founder of the Gray Panthers, who implored people: "Speak your mind—even if your voice shakes."

Elecampane *(Inula helenium)*

Grief is a watery thing that works its way into the lungs, moving downward. When the waters become stagnant, infection can set in.

Since early childhood, I have struggled with asthma and frequent bouts of bronchitis, born of grief breathed in and pushed down deep. My great-grandmother died on Christmas Eve when I was five months old. She had a long history of having breathing problems when she became emotional. And she also had a long history of drinking—perhaps to dull her senses. She was a psychically sensitive, college-educated widow living in conservative suburban upstate New York. Her mother's people came to Wisconsin from County Roscommon during the Great Hunger, and from her mother, she inherited the Sight.

I shared a strange bond with her. I was supposed to meet her the day she died, but I had bronchitis, so my mother did not take me to see her. Months later, my mother saw her ghost move my crib across the bedroom.

I inherited her patterns of breathing. I stuffed down grief and let it fill my lungs until I could not breathe. When it overflowed, I would swallow it and experience horrible gas and indigestion. When it got bad enough, I would throw up, which allowed me to breathe again.

Sensitive to the world, I worried from an early age about endangered species and nuclear war. I was a melancholy, otherworldly child, and a depressed teenager. I felt like I lived in a drowning world and could only pull more of its water into my lungs. My interpretation of Catholic theology, one quite independent of the interpretation I was taught, led me to believe that by taking that grief into myself I could somehow transmute it. The struggle for breath coupled with that theology served to alienate me from my body. And as an adult, I made a profession of being a carrier of other people's stories of suffering.

To recap a story I tell in the introduction to this book: In December of 2005, a few weeks after returning from gathering stories of torture, displacement, and the loss of land and culture in Oaxaca in the south of Mexico, I developed severe bronchitis that had me bedridden on New Year's Eve. A chance phone call that day from a perceptive herbalist I had met at a party the night I returned from Oaxaca resulted in my introduction to Elecampane—a medicine that reaches deep into the lungs and gets things moving again, releasing and cleansing buried grief just as it brings up old, infected mucus.

In *The Earthwise Herbal,* Matthew Wood writes, "Elecampane is a warming, stimulant, pungent, aromatic bitter that permeates the bronchial tree. It resolves bacterial infection, reducing heavy, thick, green mucus down to yellow and eventually to white or clear mucus. It is specific to yellow and green mucus, indicating bacterial infection. The removal of the layer of old, adhesive mucus allows for the secretion of a new layer of thin, clear mucus that is impregnated with immune factors. Meanwhile, the bitters protect the stomach against indigestion caused by mucus that is swallowed. Very typically, the person needing elecampane (often a child) swallows the mucus." Wood, of course, is describing—word for word—the pattern of disease I had developed.

I still remember the warm zing of the first drops of Elecampane tincture on my tongue that winter. The day after I started taking Elecampane, I was breathing well enough to take my dog on a long hike through the Bangor City Forest—the very place where, six months later, the *Usnea* lichen would begin to speak to me, claiming me as its own, bringing me deeper into relationship with the wild and beginning to lead me on the path of becoming an herbalist in my own right. Elecampane gave me my breath, and my breath brought me into my body, allowing me to begin to move and transform it, coming into the world in a new way.

Elecampane takes both its common name and its Latin name *(Inula helenium)* from the legend of Helen of Troy. Wood writes, "The legend is that when Helen was kidnapped by Paris, the plant sprang up from where her tears fell. Afterward the plant was known as 'Heart of the Campagna'— elecampane." Wood notes that the plant is indicated for a person who has been "torn away from [their] home, causing grief and suffering." I believe that the plant is also often indicated for those who have never felt at home in their surroundings to begin with.

It is a familiar archetype: the bookish, asthmatic child whose imagination is captivated by stories of other worlds that sound more like home than this one. At once distant and emotionally sensitive. At times deeply empathetic and perceptive, and at other times, completely oblivious to social norms and cues. Asthma, in these cases, is often closely associated with social anxiety. Breath is a tenuous thread barely keeping the child present in this reality.

In another time and place, such a child might be called "fey"—perhaps a changeling, a faerie child left in place of a stolen human one. And indeed,

Elecampane is a plant strongly associated with the faerie realm. In England, it was once commonly known as Elf Dock.

Such feelings of being born into the wrong world and the wrong body can linger into adulthood. And by the time such a child has become an adult, they have often internalized a lifetime of stories about being broken, powerless, and insufficient, eroding confidence. This can lead to an attempt to deny and suppress the sensitivity and vision that are the core of such a person's identity. More emotion pushed down into the lungs, continuing the pattern of illness. This may suggest the plant's possible historical use to treat *elfshot*, which Wood describes as "wasting and preoccupation caused by being shot by an elfin arrowhead."

At the time that I was introduced to Elecampane, I was emerging from a period of my life in which I had tried to suppress my imagination and my spirituality to gain acceptance in relationships and in the culture around me. This meant denying fundamental aspects of both my childhood and adult experiences.

Elecampane can be a powerful ally in bringing gifts from the Otherworld—wisdom obtained through grief—back into this world, integrating spiritual awareness with physical reality and bringing the spirit into the body. Breath is powerful for altering consciousness, and restoring the fluidity of breath can help someone to make the transition between different levels of reality more fluid.

Just as Elecampane works at the physical level to resolve the associated respiratory disease, the plant can also help such a person bring the gifts gained from a lifetime of gazing into other realms more fully into this world, gaining confidence and stepping into power. Elecampane brings moisture up from damp soil to feed a bright yellow flower that grows high above the ground and invites us to choose to blossom in that same way.

For me, that choice involved coming more fully into my body and into this world without denying the reality of the music I heard from the other side of the veil. It meant allowing the Pagan concept of a living earth that I professed to become real and embodied by listening to the forest and working with plants to bring healing to others and to myself.

Elecampane gave me my breath. My breath gave me life.

Bear Medicines: Skunk Cabbage, Osha, and Angelica

When Bears stir in spring, they dig their medicine roots—which Matthew Wood notes are "brown, furry, pungent, and oily," like bears themselves. Wherever people and bears live in proximity, humans have traditionally followed suit, digging and decocting those same roots. And they have told stories of people who married those strange dark giants who rear up on two legs and whose skinned bodies look human.

The Bear medicines all serve to facilitate the movement from darkness and stillness into motion and light. Their bitterness grounds us into our bodies, their heady aromatic scents melt tension to allow the blood stirred by their heat to move through the body.

Let's delve into their individual natures:

Eastern Skunk Cabbage *(Symplocarpus foetidus/Dracontium foetidus)* is the first plant to poke its head through the ground in the swamps of New England, budding just before bears come out of their dens. It melts the ice and snow around it by generating heat through a chemical process remarkably similar to that used by hibernating animals to raise their temperature as they rouse from sleep. Depending on how many acorns are left on the ground, Eastern Skunk Cabbage will make up somewhere between fifty percent and ninety-nine percent of a black bear's diet in New England in early spring.

Skunk Cabbage is perhaps best known as a respiratory medicine. The 1898 edition of the *American Dispensatory* describes Eastern Skunk Cabbage root as "a stimulant, exerting expectorant." Just as the plant's contractile roots reach deep into swampy soils to drink up moisture, the root as a medicine brings up excess mucous from deep in the lungs.

It has other ways of addressing what we hold deep below as well. Eastern Skunk Cabbage contains 5-hydroxytryptamine, an analogue to one of our own neurotransmitters—serotonin, which is responsible for opening sensory gating channels and encouraging synaptic branching in human nervous systems.

At low doses, the tincture of the root induces a deep sense of stillness and calm, like the waters of a vernal pool. William Cook described it as "a simple and reliable nervine, of the most innocent and effective soothing character" (1869b). At higher doses, the tincture begins to have an entheogenic effect. The world becomes more fluid. Distinctions between thought and emotion dissolve.

Tryptamines work to reorder the ways in which we process the information we get from the world. As entheogens, both Eastern Skunk Cabbage and Western Skunk Cabbage *(Lysichiton americanus)* seem to work with the integration of the rational consciousness of the brain and the emotional and transpersonal consciousness of the heart. (It's not clear whether Western Skunk Cabbage contains tryptamines, but Stephen Harrod Buhner first observed this phenomenon with a snuff made from Western Skunk Cabbage roots, and I've observed similar effects with the tincture.)

Eastern Skunk Cabbage has a strong affinity with the lungs (contemporary and traditional use as a stimulating expectorant), the heart (it is used for a "weak heart" among the Menominee Tribe of Wisconsin), and the waters that flow through our bodies (affinity for the kidneys and uterus). Thus, at commonly used medicinal doses, Eastern Skunk Cabbage will help to clear the physical manifestations of grief that gets buried in the lungs.

At large doses in the proper extraction, it begins to address such grief at a soul level through reconnection to the dreaming mind of the earth—especially when potentiated by an MAO-inhibitor such as Syrian Rue *(Peganum harmala)*. In the process, it carries a person through the grief of many lifetimes—a harrowing journey, to say the least. Like psilocybin, the serotonin in Skunk Cabbage and the harmaline in Syrian Rue are best extracted in a gently acidic menstruum, like vinegar.

In both cases, the healing work is not to be undertaken lightly—the pain released needs a container, and the journey back to the self is a journey through a world fraught with its own perils and challenges. Ecstatic methods require focus to avoid becoming purely chaotic and unleashing unintended consequences.

Eastern Skunk Cabbage can be a vehicle for traveling beneath the surface of the waters of consciousness, to encounter the source of the wound, and move through it and past it, undoing its power to shape consciousness and define identity. The perils lie in the potential of becoming so immersed in the pain and grief that the journey is never completed. But when the journey is completed, the wound is transformed from a source of pain to an opening between worlds that initiates the traveler into the compassion that comes from understanding grief and into the wellspring of healing. This wellspring lies beneath the surface; it comes from the heart of the universe and rises from the center of our heart to flow outward, blessing and transforming all worlds. Eastern Skunk Cabbage can offer an opening to the realms where such transformation is possible.

Western Skunk Cabbage *(Lysichiton americanus)* emerges in the swamps of the Pacific Coast as each of them finds its Imbolc—the point when winter has broken and spring is emerging. Its spathe is dusted with pollen at Bealtaine. Its medicine is quite similar to that of its eastern cousin, though there is a more uplifting feel to it.

Osha *(Ligusticum porter)* is perhaps the quintessential bear medicine. It is a powerful medicine that engages the senses intensely and works its way deep inside you.

Bears bring Osha to each other as a mating gift, an ursine aphrodisiac that they rub all over the other's body, its strong scent mingling within their own. The portion of the root that is closest to the surface resembles a bear's hair.

Osha's root can certainly stir human bodies, stirring and moving and oxygenating the blood, opening airways, raising heat. And yet it also has a long history of traditional use as a smudge and is also thrown on hot rocks to bring attention deep inward to address and heal the places in ourselves we have not previously been ready to face.

Osha is, however, highly endangered in the wild. If you don't have a direct relationship with someone who has been caretaking stands of the medicine over many years, I suggest instead combining Angelica, Shatavari, and Calamus to achieve similar effects.

Angelica *(Angelica archangelica* and *Angelica sylvestris)* is Osha's Northern European cousin. It has a lighter and brighter scent than the Rocky

Mountain bear medicine, bringing a gentler uplifting feeling while still stimulating digestion and circulation and inviting the lungs to take a deeper breath.

It is one of the principal food, medicine, and ritual plants of the Saami people. Angelica's hollow stems are made into flutes that accompany human voices and reindeer-hide drums in Saami traditional music. Matthew Wood suggests that the stem symbolizes the passage the shaman traverses between worlds. (Elder plays a similar role among Germanic and Slavic peoples a little to the south of the Saami homeland.)

Matthew Wood suggests Angelica as a medicine to restore hope to those too despondent to pray—an indication I have found reliable in my own practice. Stephen Buhner adds another dimension to this understanding—speaking of the use of Angelica for those who feel empty inside and have a sensation of hollowness in the middle of their chests.

The Bear medicines waken the sleeping Animal Self, awakening us into fuller presence.

Motherwort *(Leonurus cardiaca)*

In the midst of a winter rainstorm, at a time when my life was in turmoil, a woman I was just beginning to know—whom I now count as a dear *cara anam*, a friend of my soul—welcomed me in from the road with a cup of Motherwort tea. After drinking the tea, we lay beside the wood stove, speaking of selkies—the shape-shifting seal people of Irish and Scottish (and Maine and Nova Scotia) legend—and singing sweet, haunting old ballads while her young son slept nearby. I will always remember the gentle warmth of that night and the way I was able to put aside all my worries and allow myself to accept shelter and care. Every time I taste Motherwort, I feel like I am being tenderly held and nourished. It soothes my spirit deeply.

Like Damiana, Motherwort works with oxytocin to bring us into a place where we can receive affection and care and feel connection. But where Damiana stimulates the circulation, arousing us to movement, Motherwort soothes a heart that is beating too hard and too fast, allowing us to relax into presence and, sometimes, into sleep. Yet Motherwort will also just as easily nourish and revive a weary heart.

Motherwort reminds us that *mother* is a verb that means to give life and to love and care for that life unconditionally. It is the hand of the God Self reaching down to replenish and settle the waters of the Cauldron of Motion.

As I mentioned earlier, regarding the Cauldron of Motion, Motherwort is especially indicated where sudden surges of emotion bring heat, blood, and redness rising to the head and seek release in hot tears. I have sometimes even been able to visually observe the process of that blood flushing the neck and the face, and then, with a few drops of Motherwort, draining back down.

This downward direction of the blood flow is a property of many of the bitter mints that act on the nervous system—Motherwort, Lemon Balm, Skullcap, Wood Betony, though each does so in subtly different ways. Lemon Balm calms flashes of anger and also helps when too much sun makes someone irritable. Skullcap brings blood flow from an overactive brain down to the abdomen. And Wood Betony anchors all three selves firmly in the solar plexus to protect us from outside influences and ground us in the here and now.

Psilocybe *(Psilocybe cubensis)*

A few winters ago, I was invited to take part in another culture's medicine ceremony. The spirit of the plant we were working with told me that I was welcome to partake in the ceremony but that my people once had a similar ritual of their own.

The plant spirit called in my ancestors who showed me a vision of a man in a stone chamber wrapped in furs, playing the *bodhrán* while people sat around a fire, singing, and passing around a bowl of a purplish liquid I recognized as a tea made from *Psilocybe* mushrooms.

Several months later, I found myself standing atop a hill in a ring of Oaks planted by a bard of my tradition who had died young decades ago. I was there praying to understand how to dedicate my life to the living world without courting a similar death.

I had a vision of the queen of the Otherworld standing before me, and then I once again saw a dark stone chamber. This chamber was smaller, the size of one man's tomb, and I saw myself lying there wrapped in a Bear skin, completely still with my hands on my chest while a woman poured that same mushroom tea into my mouth and then left and sealed the chamber.

The queen told me that Bears spend nine months walking the earth and three months sleeping beneath it, listening to the songs of roots and mycelia and buried bones. She said that once upon a time, men who were pledged to her did the same—spending the dark months of the year in a continuous dreaming state brought on by being continuously fed bone broth and mushroom tea and the bright months bringing the visions incubated there to life. (An inversion of the year that followed our conception, when we spent nine months in the womb and three months in this world, learning its ways.)

She said that this was not possible in the world as it is, but that I should do what I could to follow suit in ways that fit this time and place: making the dark of the year an inward time as best I could, working with small doses of the mushrooms throughout the season and larger doses when I was in need of a more powerful vision and could carve out the time and space.

Erynn Rowan Laurie tells us that the *filidh* used periods of "incubatory darkness" to cultivate states of poetic ecstasy, and she and Timothy White provide evidence that they may have used the *Amanita muscaria* mushroom as well.

Psilocybe semilanceata is ubiquitous in Irish pastures as Samhain approaches. Nobody knows for certain how long this has been true. The dominant theory in the mycological world is that the mushroom arrived in Ireland from North America sometime in the past two centuries, but this is based on a lack of documentation of the species there prior to 1925. The absence of documentation doesn't necessarily mean the absence of the mushroom—people would have been unlikely to tell outsiders about such a medicine if they did, indeed, work with it. Some theorize that *Psilocybe* mushrooms may have been used in the *teach alais,* the sweat house. There is only the lightest bit of circumstantial evidence that this may be true, but it is consistent with the visions I was shown, which predated my reading Laurie's work and my reading about the *teach alais* by several years.

Regardless of whether they were used historically as a ritual medicine outside the places in Mexico where we have information about their traditional use, the many mushrooms of the *Psilocybe* genus make more sense as a visionary medicine for people today than *Amanita muscaria* does. *Amanita muscaria* can be toxic, is hard on the liver, and can easily and disastrously be misidentified. *Psilocybe* mushrooms are far gentler.

Speaking of plants like Dandelion and Plantain—plants that tend to follow the path of civilization's spread and tend to provide safe, gentle, but profound medicine—jim mcdonald says that there are certain plants whose habitat is the places where people live. One could say something similar about *Psilocybe* mushrooms: they love pastures created by people and live-stock, with many species favoring grasses whose roots are nourished by Cow manure and Sheep manure. They are gentler with most people than most other psychedelic medicines, though the journeys they bring you on, especially at high doses, can still be quite intense.

I think of them as showing up at civilization's edge as an antidote to civilization's mental poisons. A recent study done in London found that people with moderate depression given a regimen of meditation and psilocybin (one of the two primary serotonergic alkaloids in *Psilocybe* mushrooms) in addition to experiencing relief from their depression experienced a decreased willingness to accept the dictates of illegitimate authority and an increased sense of connection to nature. It is worth noting that *Psilocybe semilanceata*'s common name, Liberty Cap, is connected with its cap's resemblance to the caps worn by French revolutionaries in the late eighteenth century. Whether the mushroom was named for the cap or the cap was meant to represent the mushroom is a mystery.

Researchers are a bit mystified about the way in which psilocybin relieves depression. Most modern antidepressants work by slowing the reuptake of neurotransmitters to make them last longer. Psilocybin does not. It does act on serotonin (and dopamine) receptors, but in idiosyncratic ways more similar to those of the brain of a child learning new things or a person from the city brought into the wilderness. Rather than directly relieving the symptoms of depression, it seems to give people a new perspective on the things that are making them depressed.

One-time large doses of psilocybin have proven effective in shifting the anxiety and depression of people who have been diagnosed with terminal illness when those people are given guidance and a safe setting. Those shifts seem to be permanent, with people still showing positive effects from the treatment six months later. I suspect the shifts would be even more profound if the therapy were administered in a forest instead of a hospital room.

Psilocybe is undoubtedly an Otherworld medicine. It is the fruiting body of a web of connections that runs underground and feeds off the nutrients released by the decay of things that have died. It is no wonder that it facilitates a sense of connection with the living world.

The first time I worked with these mushrooms, I fasted for a day, took one-eighth of an ounce of dried *Psilocybe cubensis* mushrooms, and went into the woods with a trusted friend. I had a vision of the way the roots of all the plants intertwined and were linked together by the mycelial threads of mushrooms and felt like I could tap into the mind of the forest that this web represented—it would be at least fifteen years after that before I learned that this vision was scientifically accurate. I felt myself briefly shape-shift into the body of a Deer and nibble on the buds and tips of tree branches. Then I came back into my own body and was shown the ways in which my college campus was also an ecology of consciousness and found myself feeling deep empathy for people I had previously distrusted or disliked. It changed my experience of the world profoundly.

I don't recommend trying a dose that large without an experienced guide, a lot of preparation, and a plan for integrating what you learn.

Microdosing with *Psilocybe* mushrooms has been growing in popularity both as a way of managing depression and as a way of increasing creativity. I have seen it help people accomplish both goals, but I offer several caveats. If you are taking *Psilocybe* mushrooms to address depression but you have been living an unexamined life, you may for a time get more depressed, because the medicine invites you to look at what dwells beneath the surface of your consciousness. But if you do the work of trying to engage the questions the medicine brings to the surface, it will help you find ways of answering those questions that you might not otherwise have imagined. And if you are taking *Psilocybe* because you want to write better advertising jingles for toothpaste, it might help you to do that at first, but it's likely that it will eventually make you begin to question why you are writing stupid songs about toothpaste instead of songs about the things that make you feel alive. If you are taking the mushrooms so you can make more creative arguments to defend your client's oil pipeline, expect some nightmares. Parts of corporate America are infatuated with psychedelic microdosing right about now, but wild medicines are not easily harnessed or safely appropriated for furthering the goals of this civilization.

My preferred method of microdosing is to make an oxymel by filling a jar to the top with dried mushrooms (I personally favor *Psilocybe cubensis*) and macerating them in a combination of two-thirds vinegar and one-third honey. The vinegar, being acidic, helps to extract the psilocybin and psilocyin, which are alkaline, and the honey helps to preserve the preparation. Stored in a cool, dark place it has a shelf life of about a year in a New England climate. I recommend starting with a dose of three to five drops a day. Once you are used to the way the medicine feels, you can try slightly higher doses, titrating upward, before spending time in the forest or beneath the stars. Five milliliters is about the threshold at which I start to notice visual shifts, but I am a giant and have worked with the medicine for a long time, so I don't recommend doing anything that requires focused attention after taking more than one milliliter of the oxymel until you know how the medicine works in your particular body.

Psilocybe is a profound medicine for our times. And like all profound medicines, it needs to be approached with caution and respect.

Nettles *(Urtica dioica)*

I will end with a common plant, one quite different from the other medicines I have spoken of here. Nettles are at once nourishing and purifying, a perfect herb for helping the body navigate the transition from winter to spring, when they are one of the first wild greens present in abundance. I give them not as a drop dose tincture but as a tea or a food (and sometimes use them to sting myself, but we will get to that in a bit).

Nettle leaf soup, made with cream and butter, and sometimes seaweed, has nourished people in Ireland for thousands of years. Nettles are astoundingly nutritious. They contain more than three times as much protein and more than seventy-five times as much iron as Wheat or Barley and are also rich in calcium, magnesium, potassium, and vitamin C. The milk fat in the cream and butter in the soup aids in the absorption of many of those nutrients. Seaweed would add even more minerals.

Legend tells us that St. Colm Cille, the "Dove of the Church," exiled from Ireland to the island of Iona, was out walking one fine spring day and saw an old woman gathering Nettles. He asked her why she was doing this, and she told him that she mostly survived on Nettle soup. He then vowed to eat nothing but Nettle soup himself. A concerned monk convinced Colm Cille to allow him to prepare the soup, though, and secretly added broth to it each day.

If I were to put a client on a mono-diet, bone broth with Nettles would absolutely be my first choice. So too for my ancestors. Winter in the Irish countryside was traditionally a time of long nights spent around peat fires, taking shelter from the wind and the rain. When spring came, Nettle soup helped get the blood moving again. Irish folklorist Niall Mac Coitir writes: "Nettle was considered to be good for purifying the blood, and it was widely believed in Ireland that taking three meals of Nettles in May guarded against illness for the next year" (2017).

We now know, of course, that Nettles help the liver build blood proteins while helping the kidneys remove excess proteins (including metabolic wastes and allergens) from the blood—making them both a blood builder and a blood cleanser in a much more literal way than we usually mean when we use such terms. (It is also an amazing hemostatic herb, helping to staunch blood loss.) Dr. Kenneth Proefrock notes that thinking and worrying are metabolic activities that produce a significant amount of proteinaceous waste.

Mac Coitir adds, "In west Galway, the man of the house would go out on May Eve and gather a handful of nettles. The nettles were pressed, and everyone in the house would drink a mouthful of the juice to 'keep a good fire in them' the rest of the year." That particular turn of phrase, "keep a good fire in them" suggests Nettles role in bringing motion back to the middle cauldron. It also reflects an understanding of the way that Nettles both help to fuel our metabolic fires and clear their "ash" in order to keep them burning cleanly.

Nettles certainly get the blood flowing when they sting! There is a popular saying in Gaeilge—*Neantóg a dhóigh mé agus cupóg a leigheas mé:* "Nettle burned me, and Dock cured me." Nettles and Dock often grow side by side, and a poultice of Dock leaves helps bring down the heat and intensity of a Nettle sting. But not everyone wants to avoid Nettle stings! Because they do get the blood flowing, Nettle stings are a tried and true remedy for arthritis and gout. I have also found them a great remedy for the lethargy and depression that linger longer into springtime from winter than feels right. It is a powerful shock of electricity that can waken a nervous system or shock it into the present moment. A few drops of Lobelia will make the body even more receptive, and a few drops of Prickly Ash can bring a complementary stimulation and help the current move more efficiently through the body.

Mac Coitir reports another Irish Nettle tradition: "In southern parts of County Cork, May Eve was known as 'Nettlemas Night,' when boys would parade the streets with large bunches of Nettles, stinging their playmates and occasionally unfortunate passersby who got too close. Girls would join in too, stinging their lovers or boys for whom they held affection." Nettle stings bring an intense sensation and a rush of energy. If the Nettle leaves are a fitting medicine for the spring equinox, the Nettle sting certainly has a fitting place in youthful rites at Lá Bealtaine, with all their wild innocence.

Not all of Nettle's associations in Ireland are quite so joyful. During the An Gorta Mór, the Great Hunger, in the 1840s a million Irish died of starvation and disease and a million more fled for England or Canada or the United States or were shipped as prisoners to Australia—all while the occupying British continued to export thousands of shiploads of food grown on Irish soil to London and Liverpool and Glasgow.

Even today, the landscape in the West of Ireland is marked by the foundations of tumbledown cottages—remnants of that period—now grown over with Nettles. So common is the sight, that examples of the use of the word *neantóga* include *tá neantóga san áit a raibh an teach tráth* and *tá neantóga mar a raibh an teach tráth*—two ways of saying "there are Nettles where the house once was."

But Nettles also represent resilience. Few people know that the Great Hunger was in part a long-term consequence of the British campaign of deforestation that all but eradicated Ireland's great Oak and Hazel forests, depriving people of the Deer and Boar they once hunted and the Hazelnuts they once gathered. This deforestation also silted the streams where Salmon once swam and let the wind and rain sweep the soil into the sea. This soil depletion made Ireland's small farms especially susceptible to disasters like the blight that struck the potatoes in the 1840s. Nettles are famous for their ability to grow in and restore fertility to poor soils. Along with seaweed, they are one of the wild foods that kept many alive through the Great Hunger.

Peadar Kearney, an Irish songwriter born a generation later saw the spirit of Ireland as an old woman gathering Nettles while remembering the glories and mourning the loss of Irish men who had died in the country's many uprisings.

'Twas down by the glenside,
I met an old woman,
A-plucking young nettles,
Nor thought I was coming;

I listened awhile
To the song she was humming,
"Glory O, glory O,
To the Bold Fenian men!"

'Tis fifty long years
since I saw the moon beaming
And strong manly forms,
Their eyes with hope gleaming
I see them again
Sure, through all my days dreaming,
"Glory O, glory O,
To the Bold Fenian men!"

The Fenians were rebels who took their name from the Fianna, bands of warriors who lived in the forest, serving no one chieftain or province, but instead defending the land and the people. They were also trained as ecstatic poets and the visions they experienced in the forest would guide their actions in protecting the vulnerable. The first Fianna were trained by Fionn mac Cumhail, a warrior who had gained wisdom in his youth by accidentally eating the first bit of oil that splattered from the body of the Salmon from the Otherworld Well that his Druid teacher had caught and asked him to prepare.

In Kearney's time, another generation of Fenians rose up and won independence for all but the North of Ireland in Na Cogadh na Saoirse (the War of Freedom). He fought among them and wrote the national anthem for the Irish Republic. The Republic the former Fenian soldiers formed emerged on an island ecologically devastated by centuries of intensive occupation and exploitation. Perhaps if left to do their work, the Nettles will, in time, regenerate the land that so many generations fought to see free.

Rain seeps
through cracks
in stone foundations,

sprouting mushrooms
in empty corners
of musty rooms,

cool and dark
like the forest
that stood there

before
the first stones
were laid.

ROOTING IN THE LIVING WORLD

All medicines and all magic are rooted in cosmologies, stories about the nature of the world that are held at a level deeper then belief, things we know about life and about the world that we know all the way down to our bones. They shape the intention with which we work, often in invisible ways.

Like most Western and Westernized people, I grew up in a culture whose cosmology clashes with my own deepest truth. Our society's views—that the world is inert and the body is a machine—exist inside us, alongside the older, truer things our bodies know. This can make it challenging to trust yourself and to trust the plants and to trust the living earth. To shift this, it is helpful to engage in small ritual practices that reorient the Animal Self in time, space, and ecological community and help the Human Self develop new stories and symbols for interpreting and describing the world.

To work with Plant Allies, it is necessary to ally yourself as well with the waters of the world around you, the ancestral memories held in your bones, and the mind and spirit of the land itself. This work will be particular to you, to your lineage, and to the place that you are in.

You do not have to make a pilgrimage to a forest in your ancestral homeland or spend a year living in a yurt, listening to Coyotes and Owls sing you to sleep—though for those who can, I highly recommend these kinds of immersive, transformative experiences. There are simple things you can do that will enrich and enchant your life and connect you more deeply with the living world the plants are part of. I will break them down into four categories: connecting with your ancestors, marking seasonal shifts, honoring the source of the water you drink, and making a devotional relationship with a tree.

Connecting with Your Ancestors

Every animist culture that I am aware of honors its ancestors. And all of us are descended from animist cultures. Our neglected ancestors want to help us remember what they knew of the world.

Much has been written in recent years about ancestral trauma: about how traumatic experiences can change our DNA and how the impacts of trauma are thus passed down from one generation to the next. But if this is true (and it most definitely is) and if pleasure and joy and love shift our biochemistry as profoundly as sorrow and pain do (and they absolutely do), then aren't blessings and resilience also a part of our inheritance?

If you don't have the benefit of growing up in a living animist culture, one way to reorient to the world is to reach to the last ancestors who you are aware of who had an intact relationship with the living world around them. If you know your genealogy, look into the history and culture of the place where the oldest ancestors you are aware of lived, and trace that history back far enough to find what remnants exist of the customs and language and stories of people who experienced the world as alive and lived lives guided by the rhythms of the sun, the moon, the stars, and the earth. DNA tests can provide useful and intriguing information that might correct misremembered family origin stories or fill in gaps in information, but there are, of course, huge privacy concerns with them. If you don't know who your ancestors were, spend some time looking at photographs of different regions of the world and notice where you feel a resonance.

Make a small altar honoring your ancestors somewhere in your home. It can be simple to begin with: a picture or an object connected with the part of the world where they lived, a glass or cup to fill with water, and a small plate on which to make food offerings. Research the foods of that part of the world. Once a week, prepare one of those foods and sit down at the altar, giving a portion to the ancestors and a portion to yourself (if you eat with your family, it might be good to have an ancestor altar or altars in the room where you eat). Let your senses take in the scents and flavors and textures of the food and hold the intention of letting them awaken in you the things your ancestors would like for you to remember.

Next, begin to look to language as a way of connecting with your ancestors. Sound resonates throughout our fascia and in our bones, and our bodies remember it deeply. From an early age, every time I have heard Irish Gaeilge spoken or sung (which, I think, may even have happened when my grandparents took me to meet my Great Uncle Jigs, who played the squeezebox and was the first musician and first Irish speaker I ever met), I have felt myself shift into a different way of seeing the world, even without understanding a single word being spoken. The way words vibrate our vocal chords and echo in our chests when we speak or sing them also awakens ancestral memory in our bodies. I still have only enough Irish Gaeilge to make strange prayers and express stranger endearments, but speaking those words and phrases I have brings the feeling of my ancestors standing with me.

I recommend beginning with learning to say "thank you" in that language. The great Christian mystic Meister Eckhart said, "If the only prayer you said was 'thank you,' that would be enough." I know the Divine by different names than he did, but gratitude is also the place where all my prayers begin. When I give thanks for my own life and the lives of my human and wild kin, I come into knowing my place in the world, and from there I can find the courses of action that will bring the greatest blessing to the community of life.

Learn what the words literally mean. *Go raibh míle maith agat* is the Irish way of saying "Thank you very much," but it literally means "may a thousand good things come toward you." Knowing that, when I speak the words, I feel the winds and currents that will carry all those good things to the person whose happiness I am praying for as I express my gratitude. (Sometimes that person is an Oak or a Stag or a stone.)

Pay careful attention to everything you feel when you speak these words.

Once you have mastered a few simple phrases, see if you can learn a poem or a song that is meaningful to you in that language. A few years before he became poet laureate of the United States, I heard Robert Pinsky speak about how reading a poem aloud is an intimate act that connects you with everyone else who has ever read that poem aloud, because you are all shaping the column of breath within your bodies in the same way.

If you can, find the oldest stories available that are associated with your ancestors and tell them to people you love on dark winter nights. Then pay careful attention to your dreams.

Marking the Seasons

As I said when writing about the Cauldron of Motion, my teacher, Cornelia Benavidez, recently reminded me that people around the world have always marked seasonal changes and the cycles of the sun, the moon, and the stars with shared work, feasting, and ritual. What do you do if you don't already mark these cycles in your life?

One thing you can do is look to your ancestral traditions of marking the seasons—but the seasons where you are might be different from the seasons where your ancestors lived. It is still well worth looking for elements of their seasonal rituals that might be incorporated into your own, this will deepen your connection with them.

The best thing to do is to make a point of walking in the same forest once a week, every week for a year. Keep track of the changes you feel in your body and the changes you witness in the forest and look up (or, better yet, observe) what is happening with the sun, the moon, the stars, and the weather. Notice the big turning points, when changes in your body and changes in the land quicken. These will be the points you will choose for next year's celebration. Note as many of the changes taking place in these times as you can, and look for the energetic nature of the shifts the pattern of signs indicates.

The following year, during each of those major turning points, invite friends to do some work with you outdoors that is fitting for the season and then share a meal of seasonal, local food. Do this every year.

Honoring the Waters

Water is central to my cosmology and to the cosmology of my ancestors, as this book has made clear. Water is also what we are mostly made of and what plants are mostly made of.

Find out where the water you drink comes from. Once a week, if it is nearby—and once a season, if it is far from you—bring a simple offering to the water and say "thank you" in one of your ancestral languages. I personally favor whiskey, honey, and milk as offerings.

Find a place where there is wild water near you. Once a week spend at least half an hour gazing at the water and bringing your focus back to the sight and sound of the water every time your attention wanders. Find out what watershed you live in—the place where the water that falls on the ground flows to. Regularly bring offerings of purifying herbs to that water. Find out what threatens the health of the waters of your home and find what you can do to protect and restore them.

Begin each day with a glass of water and the words "thank you."

Making a Devotional Relationship with a Tree

Trees are the memory keepers of the land. The shape of their trunks shows the way the wind blows over years, decades, or even centuries. Their wood holds the memory of sunlight and rainfall. Their roots tap in to the mycorrhizal network that is the mind of the forest, and their bodies feel and remember the changes in the chemical and photic and electromagnetic conversations happening across the braided tendrils of that sylvan consciousness.

Find the oldest tree within easy travel of your home. Once a week bring an offering to the tree. Sit with it and say "thank you." Then become quiet and lean against the tree, letting your body feel its support. Let your feet feel the ground beneath you—and the way the roots run beneath them. Notice the sensations and emotions you feel. And the dreams you have that night.

Find stories and poems about the species of tree that your tree belongs to. Notice which ones remind you of your tree and which ones do not. Read the ones that resonate aloud to your tree.

If you find a fallen leaf beneath your tree, you might put it under your pillow and notice what you dream. If you find a fallen branch, you might place it on an altar or hang it over your bed. Watch the changes in your tree over the course of the year.

Find out what your tree needs to thrive, and do your best to help create those conditions. Find out what that species of tree needs to thrive in the forests around you, and do what you can to protect and nurture all of your tree's kin.

Reciprocity is at the heart of animist relationships with the living world. Robin Wall Kimmerer writes, "Action on behalf of life transforms. Because the relationship between self and the world is reciprocal, it is not a question of first getting enlightened or saved and then acting. As we work to heal the earth, the earth heals us."

Such an ethic of reciprocity is rare in our culture, but in England and Wales, it lives on in the custom of wassailing. If there are fruit trees or fruit bushes near you, consider wassailing them when winter comes. Those who are familiar with the custom tend to associate it with the solstice or Twelfth Night, but in parts of Cornwall and the English West Country, wassailing season extends into late January. Wassailing is the custom of bringing offerings of cider and song to Apple trees in hopes of an abundant harvest the following autumn.

I learned years ago from Stephen Buhner that Apple trees get drunk on their own fermented fruit, becoming lulled into a sleep that protects them through the cold winter. I think of traditions of not harvesting any of the fruit that was on the trees or on the ground after Samhain, and wonder if that began in acknowledgment not only of the needs of Deer but also the needs of Apple trees. I think also of the thaws that sometimes come in January in many northern climes and wonder if cider and song may help an Apple tree waking before its time to sink back into dreaming.

Certainly, wassailing aids human hearts in dreaming their way back into a reciprocal relationship with their plant kin.

And in return, our plant kin help us dream our way back into wholeness.

The mountain is wreathed
by the smoke of burning forests

and across the ocean
pilots prepare
to set cities aflame.

But in this same world,
Bears crash through
thickets of huckleberries,
Salmon prepare for
their journey back
to the streams where
they were born,

and in autumn
Bears drag
the carcasses of Salmon
into the forest

where they
rot into the topsoil

and are reborn
as Cedar
and Trillium
and Wild Ginger.

Long ago
someone wrote

"Empires
rise and fall
but the mountains
and rivers
remain."

It is only because
we have forgotten

that we are dancing mountains
and flowing rivers

that we think
that the world
might end.

EPILOGUE

The Age of Burning Forests

F orests are burning as I write.

From Siberia to the Amazon to Angola to Indonesia, the smoke and flames are visible from space. The temperate rainforests I once called home on North America's Pacific Coast are burning, too. As they burn, so does an essential part of the memory and knowledge of who we are.

As they burn, a pandemic rages, which brings fire into the airways and blood vessels of millions, changing their lives permanently, as it has mine, or ending their lives completely.

More than ever, we need to remember our kinship with the forest. Humans evolved in forests and savannahs, shaped by the living world around us.

Our senses and our sensory processing evolved to favor subtle information about the bodies and presence of people and animals and plants. Living in small, tight-knit human communities that were woven in interdependent relationships with the other-than-human life around them, our ancestors possessed an orientation toward connection that they passed down to us. When we find comfort in the scent of the skin of someone we love, the night chorus of frogs, the sound of leaves rustling in the wind, we are experiencing the somatic and emotional echoes of what it meant for our ancestors to live in a world they experienced as alive and always speaking to them.

Our nervous and endocrine systems involved responding to chemical signals from plants that arrived in the air our ancestors breathed, the water they drank, the brush of leaf and petal against skin. We feel it still when the wind brings us the scent of Cottonwood in springtime, when we walk among Cedars after a summer rainstorm, and when we breathe in the sweet, pungent perfume of fallen Apples among fallen leaves in autumn.

Is it any wonder that in lives where we rarely have the opportunity to be deeply present to each other and to a wild world that seems to recede further and further from us, so many of us live lives where we hunger voraciously for levels of meaning and connection that seem to elude us, and so many of us struggle with anxiety, terror, numbness, grief, and rage?

Coming home to the knowledge of who we are depends on reconnecting with the living world around us.

The forest reminds us who we are.

Remembering who we are, we feel our kinship for the forest, and understand that our lives are intertwined.

So it has been in my life. So it can be in yours. So it must be in the lives of people around the world if the forest and the people are to live.

BIBLIOGRAPHY

Anderson, Cora. 2010. *Fifty Years in the Feri Tradition*. Portland, OR: Harpy Books.

Anderson, Victor H., and Cora Anderson. 2004. *Etheric Anatomy: The Three Selves and Astral Travel*. Albany, CA: Acorn Guild Press.

Artisson, Robin. 2018. *An Carow Gwyn: Sorcery and the Ancient Fayerie Faith*. Bangor, ME: Black Malkin Press.

Benavidez, Cornelia, Victor H. Anderson, and Cora Anderson. 2017. *Victor H. Anderson: An American Shaman*. Stafford, England: Megalithica Book.

Blackie, Sharon. 2019. *If Women Rose Rooted: A Life-Changing Journey to Authenticity and Belonging*. Tewkesbury, England: September Publishing.

Buhner, Stephen Harrod. 1998. *Sacred and Herbal Healing Beers: The Secrets of Ancient Fermentation*. Boulder, CO: Siris Books.

———. 2004. *The Secret Teachings of Plants: The Intelligence of the Heart in the Direct Perception of Nature*. Rochester, VT: Bear.

———. 2014. *Plant Intelligence and the Imaginal Realm: Beyond the Doors of Perception into the Dreaming Earth*. Rochester, VT: Bear.

Child, Francis James. n.d. "37A: Thomas Rymer." The Child Ballads: 37. Thomas Rymer. www.sacred-texts.com/neu/eng/child/ch037.htm.

Cook, William. 1869a. "Cimicifuga Racemosa. Black Cohosh, Rattleroot." In *The Physio-medical Dispensatory: A Treatise on Therapeutics, Materia Medica, and Pharmacy, in Accordance with the Principles of Physiological Medication*. Cincinnati. Available online at Henriette's Herbal Homepage. www.henriettes-herb.com /eclectic/cook/cimicifuga_racemosa.htm.

———. 1869b. "Symplocarpus Foetidus. Skunk Cabbage." In *The Physio-medical Dispensatory: A Treatise on Therapeutics, Materia Medica, and Pharmacy, in Accordance with the Principles of Physiological Medication*. Cincinnati. Available online at Henriette's Herbal Homepage. www.henriettes-herb.com/eclectic/cook /symplocarpus_foetidus.htm.

Dharmananda, Subhuti. n.d. "Kidney Essence and the Human Body: An Exploration of Chinese Embryology." www.itmonline.org/arts/essence.htm.

Dimech, Alkistis. 2016. "Dynamics of the Occulted Body." Scarlet Imprint. May 6. https://scarletimprint.com/essays/dynamics-of-the-occulted-body.

Federici, Silvia. 2016. "In Praise of the Dancing Body." Gods and Radicals, August 22. https://godsandradicals.org/2016/08/22/in-praise-of-the-dancing-body.

Felter, Harvey Wickes, and John Uri Lloyd. 1898. "Dracontium.-Skunk-Cabbage." In *King's American Dispensatory*. Cincinnati: Ohio Valley. Available online at Henriette's Herbal Homepage. www.henriettes-herb.com/eclectic/kings /dracontium.html.

Frances, Deborah. 1996. "Crataegus: Mental and Emotional Indications." *Medical Herbalism: Journal for the Clinical Practitioner* 8, no. 3: 1, 4. http://medherb.com /materia_medica/crataegus_-_mental_and_emotional_indications.htm.

Gantz, Jeffrey. 1988. *Early Irish Myths and Sagas*. London: Penguin.

Gregory, Lady Augusta. n.d. "Visions and Beliefs in the West of Ireland." Internet Sacred Texts Archive. www.sacred-texts.com/neu/celt/vbwi.

Heaney, Seamus. 2001. *Sweeney Astray: A Version from the Irish*. London: Faber and Faber.

Hedley, Gil. n.d. "How I Fell In Love With Fat" Exploring Inner Space. https:// sensualiq.com/blogs/exploring_inner_space_files/how_i_fell_in_love_with _fat.html.

Iwersen, Julia. n.d. "Virgin Goddess." Encyclopedia. Accessed October 16, 2020. www.encyclopedia.com/environment/encyclopedias-almanacs-transcripts-and -maps/virgin-goddess.

Kearney, Peadar. n.d. "Bold Fenian Men." All Poetry. https://allpoetry.com/Bold -Fenian-Men.

Kimmerer, Robin Wall. 2020. *Braiding Sweetgrass: Indigenous Wisdom, Scientific Knowledge, and the Teachings of Plants*. New York: Penguin.

Laurie, Erynn Rowan. 2007. *Ogam: Weaving Word Wisdom*. Stafford, England: Megalithica Books.

———. n.d. "The Cauldron of Poesy." The Preserving Shrine. www.seanet.com /~inisglas/cauldronpoesy.html.

Laurie, Erynn Rowan, and Timothy White. n.d. "Speckled Snake, Brother of Birch: *Amanita Muscaria* Motifs in Celtic Legends." The Preserving Shrine. www .seanet.com/~inisglas/AmanitaArticle.pdf.

Lawrence, David Herbert, and Michael Squires. 2010. *Lady Chatterley's Lover; and A Propos of "Lady Chatterley's Lover"*. Cambridge: Cambridge University Press.

Lenihan, Edmund, and Carolyn Eve Green. 2004. *Meeting the Other Crowd: The Fairy Stories of Hidden Ireland*. New York: Jeremy P. Tarcher/Penguin.

Lifton, Robert Jay, and Richard A. Falk. 1991. *Indefensible Weapons: The Political and Psychological Case against Nuclearism*. New York: Basic Books.

Lorca, Federico García. n.d. "Theory and Play of the *Duende*." Translated by A. S. Kline. Poetry in Translation. www.poetryintranslation.com/PITBR/Spanish/LorcaDuende.php.

Mac Coitir, Niall. 2016. *Ireland's Trees: Myths, Legends and Folklore*. Cork, Ireland: Collins Press.

———. 2017. *Ireland's Wild Plants: Myths, Legends and Folklore*. Cork, Ireland: Collins Press.

Mac Coitir, Niall, and Gordon D'Arcy. 2015. *Ireland's Animals: Myths, Legends and Folklore*. Cork, Ireland: Collins Press.

Macy, Joanna, and Molly Young Brown. 2014. *Coming Back to Life: The Updated Guide to The Work That Reconnects*. Gabriola Island, BC: New Society.

Masé, Guido. 2013. *The Wild Medicine Solution: Healing with Aromatic, Bitter, and Tonic Plants*. Rochester, VT: Healing Arts Press.

mcdonald, jim. n.d. "Herbal Properties and Actions" Herbcraft. https://herbcraft.org/properties.html.

Mickaharic, Draja. *A Century of Spells*. San Francisco: Red Wheel/Weiser, 1990.

Moriarty, John. 2006. *Invoking Ireland = Ailiu Iath n-hErend*. Dublin, Ireland: Lilliput Press.

———. 2009. *Dreamtime*. Dublin, Ireland: Lilliput Press.

Pendell, Dale. 2009a. *Pharmako/Dynamis: Stimulating Plants, Potions, and Herbcraft*. Berkeley, CA: North Atlantic Books.

———. 2009b. *Pharmako/Gnosis: Plant Teachers and the Poison Path*. Berkeley, CA: North Atlantic Books.

———. 2010. *Pharmako/Poeia: Plant Powers, Poisons, and Herbcraft*. Berkeley, CA: North Atlantic Books.

Pert, Candace B., and Deepak Chopra. *Molecules of Emotion: Why You Feel the Way You Feel*. New York: Scribner, 2003.

Reich, Wilhelm. 1973. *Ether, God, and Devil/Cosmic Superimposition*. Translated by Therese Pol. New York: Farrar, Straus and Giroux.

———. 1978. *The Function of the Orgasm: Sex-Economic Problems of Biological Energy*. Translated by Vincent R. Carfagno. New York: Pocket Books.

———. 2018. *The Mass Psychology of Fascism*. Edited by Mary Higgins and Chester M. Raphael. London, England: Souvenir Press (E & A).

Savarese, Ralph. 2014. "I Object: Autism, Empathy, and the Trope of Personification." Emory University, March 3, 2014, video, 53:55, Ralph Savarese of Grinnell College advances the notion of a much less human-centered empathy by exploring the propensity in autism to attend to objects more than people (February 19).

Schulke, Daniel A. 2005. *Viridarium Umbris: The Pleasure Garden of Shadows.* Chelmsford, UK: Xoanon Limited.

Tolf, Christine. n.d. "Flower Essences A—F." Lichenwood Herbals. Accessed November 9, 2020. www.lichenwood.com/flower-essences-a—-f.html.

Tozzi, Paolo. 2014. "Does Fascia Hold Memories?" *Journal of Bodywork and Movement Therapies* 18, no. 2: 259–65. https://doi.org/10.1016/j.jbmt.2013.11.010.

Walker, Nick. 2013. "Throw Away the Master's Tools: Liberating Ourselves from the Pathology Paradigm." Neurocosmopolitanism. August 16. https://neurocosmopolitanism.com/throw-away-the-masters-tools-liberating-ourselves-from-the-pathology-paradigm.

———. 2014a. "What Is Autism?" Neurocosmopolitanism. March 1. https://neurocosmopolitanism.com/what-is-autism.

———. 2014b. "Neurodiversity: Some Basic Terms and Definitions" Neurocosmopolitanism. September 27. https://neurocosmopolitanism.com/neurodiversity-some-basic-terms-definitions/.

Waters, Jennifer. 2015. "The Way We Are Designed: A Conversation with Gil Hedley, PhD." *Acupuncture Today* 16, no. 4. www.acupuncturetoday.com/mpacms/at/article.php?id=33012.

Weschler, Lawrence. 2015. "A Rare, Personal Look at Oliver Sacks's Early Career." *Vanity Fair.* June. www.vanityfair.com/culture/2015/04/oliver-sacks-autobiography-before-cancer.

Wilde, Lady Jane Francesca. 1888. "Ancient Legends, Mystic Charms, and Superstitions of Ireland (1888)." LibraryIreland. www.libraryireland.com/AncientLegendsSuperstitions/Contents.php.

Wilson, Peter Lamborn. 1999. *Ploughing the Clouds: The Search for Irish Soma.* San Francisco: City Lights.

Wood, Matthew. 1998. *The Book of Herbal Wisdom: Using Plants as Medicine.* Berkeley, CA: North Atlantic Books.

———. 2008. *The Earthwise Herbal: A Complete Guide to Old World Medicinal Plants.* Berkeley, CA: North Atlantic Books.

———. 2009. *The Earthwise Herbal: A Complete Guide to New World Medicinal Plants.* Berkeley, CA: North Atlantic Books.

Yeats, William Butler. 1991. *Selected Poetry.* Edited by Timothy Webb. Harmondsworth, England: Penguin.

INDEX

ABOUT THE AUTHOR

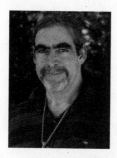 SEÁN PÁDRAIG O'DONOGHUE is an herbalist, writer, and teacher, and an initiated Priest in two traditions. He lives in the mountains of western Maine. Seán's approach to healing weaves together the insights of traditional Western herbalism and contemporary science. He regards physical, spiritual, and emotional healing as deeply intertwined.

Prior to becoming an herbalist, Seán was a political organizer in movements for peace, human rights, and global economic justice, and a freelance journalist documenting the human and ecological impacts of U.S. policies in Latin America.

He grew up near Boston, a short distance from where his great-grandparents first landed when they arrived from Ireland. Since childhood, he has been an avid student of Irish history and folklore. He graduated from Dartmouth College in 1996 with a degree in English literature and creative writing.

About North Atlantic Books

North Atlantic Books (NAB) is an independent, nonprofit publisher committed to a bold exploration of the relationships between mind, body, spirit, and nature. Founded in 1974, NAB aims to nurture a holistic view of the arts, sciences, humanities, and healing. To make a donation or to learn more about our books, authors, events, and newsletter, please visit www.northatlanticbooks.com.

North Atlantic Books is a 501(c)(3) nonprofit educational organization that promotes cross-cultural perspectives linking scientific, social, and artistic fields. To learn how you can support us, please visit our website.